CW00967681

The Babe with the Power

JOYEL MARIE

Copyright © 2024 by Joyel Marie

All rights reserved. No part of this publication may be reproduced, distributed, or transmitted in any form or by any means, including photocopying, recording, or other electronic or mechanical methods, without the prior written permission of the publisher, except in the case of brief quotations embodied in critical reviews and certain other noncommercial uses permitted by copyright law.

For permission requests, write to the author at: joyelmariebooks@gmail.com

Joyel Marie
The Babe with the Power / Joyel Marie —1st ed.

Paperback: 979-8-9903344-0-3
Hardback: 979-8-9903344-1-0
Ebook: 979-8-9903344-2-7

This book is dedicated to you, reader. May you find your power.

Contents

Preface

Labyrinth is a 1986 cult classic film by Jim Henson. It stars David Bowie as the dreamy yet menacing Goblin King and Jennifer Connelly as Sarah, a disgruntled teenager who wishes her baby half-brother would be taken away. Sarah must traverse a dangerous labyrinth to rescue her brother from the Goblin City, and each twist and turn signifies far more than what is portrayed on screen.

It was, and still is, one of my favorite films.

It turns out, however, that Jim Henson didn't know the magical metaphor he was writing when he created *Labyrinth*. And David Bowie didn't know what he was writing in the title track "(Dance) Magic Dance" when he said, "The babe with the power." I know this because I'm a bit of a fan—still today. More than my nine-year-old self watching on my living room floor eating fireballs with my best friend recording the worm with the funny accent saying 'ello on my pink plastic boombox, hoping you couldn't hear my grandmother talking in the kitchen on the cassette.

I know this because I bought the book with Jim Henson's sketches and notes on the movie. In March 1983, he drafted monsters and puzzles that evolved into the labyrinth. He didn't mention Sarah. Later, in July of that same year, his notes included the Goblin King. He still didn't know it would be a female heroine's journey. And he most certainly didn't know about the magical symbolism.

Honestly, after watching the film, I didn't either.

Jim and his director friend George Lucas didn't initially plan for Sarah to make up the whole thing in her head. But eventually, that's where the movie ended up. She built all the walls. And the point was her taking personal responsibility for herself and her life. No more blaming. All those walls. All those puzzles. Just a journey to come full circle.

We all do the same thing, don't we? Make walls and create our own pain and our own path. And we can either sit on the sand looking over at the labyrinth and not enter, for it's pretty scary. Or we can charge ahead and tear it down from the inside out.

As I tracked back through my childhood, adolescent, and adult struggles, I saw them as massive cinder blocks forming into my very own labyrinth walls. It was like Jim Henson's story was happening to *me*. I was the victim caged by these unrelenting bricks of cement. As I moved through the drafting process and the systematic excavation of my life and memories, I began to see how I, like Sarah, had played a part in building those walls. Sure, life had dealt me some challenging circumstances, but I began to see how readily I had laid the mortar between each brick and claimed the limitations as my own. Like Sarah, I realized that it was my job to tear those walls down.

No one really ever knows you. Sure, your mom or your oldest friend likely knows you the best, but they don't know what goes on with you under the skin, under the cover of the façade. Perhaps they can sense something has always been wrong, but they've never been sure exactly what. They don't know that you never really trusted them. They don't know how deep the well of darkness goes, the times you were on the verge of suicide. The have no idea how giant the labyrinth of walls you have built is or how heavy the cinderblocks are that sit on your chest. They don't know how much you resented the world, and the only way you could escape the pain was by looking at that little razor on the side of the tub.

The well is deep, my friend. And we can pull each other out if we dare to reach our hand up. Or find a monster named Hoggle or Ludo to witness our rise from the depths. Because we are better together. And they are there, should you need them.

Let me be clear. This is a memoir, a relatively chronological memoir filled with life lessons I want to share. I want to inspire those ready to heal, women in difficult work environments, and those who have generational and personal emotional trauma to heal—trauma that may not even be real but cultivated by the environment they grew up in. I want to inspire you to navigate this dark, difficult time by being yourself and finding the courage to face the labyrinth.

This book is also a call for more love and kindness. To ourselves and others and the earth. A call for more joy. We must find the quiet to see the sparkle in this dark time. To settle into our roots, buy local, reframe, and rewild ourselves. I struggled to decide if I wanted to create a self-help book instead. I've spent so much time trying to escape real life in food, the labyrinth, and self-pity. Every single thing I've ever tried to escape didn't work.

I'm also writing this during a time when I healed from compulsive overeating. I never liked the term "healing journey," but it's true. I used to feel like it implied that I was broken. *I have to admit that I'm broken?* Apparently. I think that's pretty obvious by my size, but I know of many "normal-sized" people who have a lot of food issues to heal from, too.

Geneen Roth, an author and teacher in the field of eating disorders, says, "Your relationship to food, no matter how conflicted, is the doorway to freedom." My food healing is like a purging, a death of the old me. The next chapter is blank, but not blank. I realize that we create our future based on who we think we are. Whatever the mind can conceive and believe, it achieves. Well, I spent a lifetime (thirty-eight years, to be exact) believing that I was fat. It was a long journey to discover I can have a positive relationship with my food and my body. My body is a fantastic feat of a million miracles a day.

I'm also writing this book, in part, because I have trouble expressing my spiritual beliefs, as I think many do. I thought maybe writing them down for myself would help others navigate our incredibly complex religious history and find righteousness in the boiled-down purities that all religions are supposedly based on. I was raised Catholic, spent a long time as an agnostic, then atheist, and now I call myself spiritual, but not religious. (There's a whole organization called this, but I'm not part of that either). I am open to all. I am not tied to any institution.

God is a word humans have created to define the beauty in science, nature, and the universe. I like the word Universe. God still evokes some trauma that may not yet be healed. The word God, or Lord, makes my upper lip curl, my nose crinkle, and my eyes frown. It evokes patriarchal pain specifically. Pain from wars (that are starting again), pain from institutions, and the realization that it's all based on some guy's fear of losing his power.

HIS power.

It makes me want to rip up a picture of the Pope just like Sinead O'Connor did on *Saturday Night Live*. It makes me think of little boys being molested behind the altar. I want to scream at them all. All in the name of God. So, apparently, I still have some letting go and healing to do about that little three-letter word.

I'm, of course, riddled with a bit of doubt.

No one will want to read this. Who do you think you are? You are so basic.

The mean committee in my head keeps chirping.

Go away, I clap back.

I take a deep breath and think about how dreams are gifts, and for some reason, this is what I dream and am being called to do. I want to express what I want to express. Period. If no one reads it, so be it. I want the words dripping off my fingers into this computer to wash over your eyes and brain, smooth the shoulders, make the eyes close, and put the book down to contemplate or in awe or sympathetic understanding.

And so, I think of those who taught me to recognize those thoughts of doubt. Face them, even talk to them. "Hello, doubt. What else?"

I say, "Thank you, reptilian, fear-based brain, for protecting me. But I still want to do this even if not a single person reads it. Or a million people read this, and they send me truckloads of hate mail."

Who knows? Maybe Oprah will have me on her podcast someday, or I'll take my book out of the Earlville Library someday.

Come on, hands, let's go.

Building the Walls

CHAPTER 1

Less Than Zero

We live as we dream, alone.

–GANG OF FOUR

My existence was a scandal.

And writing it will be another.

You see, my family does not talk about things. We quietly ignore them. We don't look at them. We don't lean into conflict. We don't examine. Especially the big things.

We don't talk about the dark-haired, dark-skinned girl (that's me) in a family full of blond-haired, blue-eyed Germans. We don't talk about where or who her father might be. We don't talk about her mentally ill grandmother, talking to the wall at Thanksgiving like a homeless bag lady.

Nope, we don't talk about her.

We sit there staring at our turkey and mashed potatoes with cranberry sauce. I stuff the bread and butter down deep into the corners of my mouth.

We don't talk about her toenails growing so long they curled up.

We for sure don't talk about religion or beliefs or addictions or feelings or emotions. We don't talk about how my uncle doesn't come around anymore. We don't talk about my divorce or what happened.

Nope.

We might talk a little about politics, but it's mostly kids, cars, work, football, local construction, and the new shed out back. Keep it light, robotic, serious but surface-level. So, my writing about and talking about the truth will be another scandal.

I concluded at seven years old that I must have been adopted. Not only didn't I feel a part of this family, but I also didn't feel a part of this world. I felt wrong in my body, wrong in my skin, wrong in the Catholic church, wrong in Catholic school. But I didn't know how to articulate that deep ache of not belonging. The evidence, the clear and objective evidence, was that my skin was dark brown, and everyone else was white as a sheet. It was too compelling for my seven-year-old brain.

My mother and I shared the pink room at the top of the stairs in my grandparents' house. Pink rose wallpaper, pink shag carpet, and our two pink headboards painted to hide the green plastic underneath. Our twin beds sandwiched a tiny nightstand. As we lay there one night, separated by this small chasm of space, I argued with my mom that I must be adopted.

"You are *not* adopted!"

"Then show me my birth certificate!"

Surely, this official document would hold the truth.

She sighed heavily, quietly rose, and went to the hallway closet. I sat perched on my bed, my hands gripping the white summer quilt and matching white sheets with the dainty yellow flowers. I was scared and excited. The room was dark, but the hall light cast enough of a glow to see the silhouette of my mom on the landing that split the home's two small upstairs bedrooms.

She lifted a metal fireproof file box from the closet, removed the lid, and opened a yellow envelope. She had resigned herself to giving me what I wanted but was tentative about showing it to me. My mom slid out the evidence I'd requested and handed me the manila paper with the raised seal. I held the document in my hands, studying the border before my eyes scanned the words.

Mother: Mary Ann Kerl

Father:

It was blank.

What the hell does that mean?

I probably wasn't swearing in my head at seven, but I'm sure that's generally what I was thinking.

"Well, who is my father then?"

"You're too young to understand," she replied.

And that was the answer I got until I was twenty-one, no matter how many times I asked.

As a child, all I really wanted to know was who my dad was. What did he look like? Why was he not here? What did he sound like? What was his favorite song to listen to on the radio?

My heart pined when I saw other dads with their daughters. I fantasized about Bruce Willis from *Moonlighting* adopting me. My mom and I used to watch the show together, and I loved the attention his character gave to Cybill Shepherd's. I liked his apartment, and I vaguely remember one episode where he took in a young girl in need of care. I clung to that fantasy. I imagined a mattress on the floor and him making me breakfast.

And if I couldn't have an actual father, I at least wanted an explanation of who I was. But it would be years before I got that information, years before I would learn the truth that would flood me with new rivers of shame about my real identity.

When my mom finally told me about my dad, we stood over a cheesecake she had asked me to get from the garage. Growing up we used the garage as a porch, or "Florida room." We had a permanent screen made to cover the door. There was furniture, indoor/outdoor carpet, a table in the center, a refrigerator, and a bin to store outdoor toys. Many parties and family holidays were celebrated in that garage. When my mom invited extra guests to Thanksgiving—people who had nowhere else to go—we'd overflow into the garage if the weather was nice enough.

The garage became the cold storage for winter holidays when temperatures were frigid. The Christmas cheesecake, the rolls, or the ham could be stored on the table in the garage. A high school crush once made me feel like a piece of trash for using a garage as a porch. He said he hated the Buffalo culture and people and called them lower-class citizens.

"I could never date someone who used their garage as a porch," he snarled.

That's what my family did, and I feel no shame. It's your loss, buddy. My family and friends had many happy memories out there.

I don't remember what holiday it was, but I remember the temperature being cool yet warm enough to be in the garage for a holiday get-together. Maybe it was Easter. I was home from college, and I was helping my mom get ready for company. I put the pickles and olives in crystal dishes with the little separator and then covered them with plastic wrap.

"Let's get out the maraschino cherries and cut them and put them on the cheesecake," she said.

In my memory, it was cheesecake. We've never put cherries on a cheesecake, only kuchen or some glazed pastry, so I'm not sure if my memory is failing me or if we put cherries on the cheesecake this time.

As we stood side by side, cutting and placing cherries, I asked again, "Are you ever going to tell me the story of my father?"

We didn't look at each other. We stood there staring down at that cheesecake. And she began to talk.

With a long sigh, she said, "His name was Louis."

I sucked in a small breath to keep myself from speaking, and I could feel the air tingle a bit in my lungs. This was it. I was finally going to have all the answers.

"I don't know his last name, just that he was from Puerto Rico," she continued. "I was in Toronto with my friends. We were all at the hotel bar. He told me he was on a business trip. One moment, we were in the bar at the hotel, and the next… Well, I don't remember anything after that. I don't know if he drugged me or I just had too much to drink. Either way, it was not consensual."

We shared a long pause as I absorbed what she was saying.

"That's why I'm always worried about your drinking," she admitted.

"Was he married? Did he have any other children?" I prodded.

"I don't know."

"What did the family say?" I pressed.

"I had been dating an Italian guy a few months before the trip, and I figured they assumed you were his."

She never told her friends what had happened that night. I assume she was embarrassed, but remember, we don't talk about things in this family.

No one ever asked. No one ever said anything.

She told me that when she realized she was pregnant, she was too afraid to tell her father. So she drove out to Indianapolis to see my uncle Buddy. She begged him to come home with her for moral support while she broke the news, and he did. Even though my mom had other brothers in Buffalo (she was one of six kids), she was always closest to Uncle Buddy and needed him at that moment. It's why he's my godfather.

When she got pregnant with me, she chose to live at home. She was a single mother and felt she needed the support of her family, so she lived with her parents in the house she grew up in and raised me there.

Because I grew up with my grandmother and grandfather, almost all holidays were at our 1,100-square-foot, A-frame house in a well-to-do suburb of Buffalo, New York, called East Amherst. Most houses were worth over $250,000 (now likely well over $1M), and Jim Kelly, the famous quarterback for the Buffalo Bills, allegedly lived down the road for a short period of time. University professors and other wealthy people lived in the developments around us, but we lived on one of the original roads of the area.

My mother remembers the area as rural before any developments. She would tell me stories of running in the woods when she was little. Now, it's all newer-construction homes. My grandfather bought our house when it was brand new in 1955 for $11,000.

I think a lot about my scandalous existence and the ripples it sent through that family.

My mother was a good Catholic girl who attended Catholic school, was raised by a good Catholic family, attended church every Sunday, and followed the rules. How did my mom and family handle dealing with this unwed girl who got pregnant in 1974? What fear my mom must have faced, what shame. She must have held her head down and ducked out of church as fast as she could. The fear of judgment from the family, the church, and the small community in the suburbs of Buffalo in good old Upstate New York.

I found out later that my uncle (the one who doesn't come around much anymore) said something nasty to my mom, and that's why she would always go up to her room when he came over, why he never showed up at full-family holiday events. I can only imagine what was said since she has never told me. But of course, you know how they dealt with this. They put their heads down, didn't talk about it, and kept on keepin' on.

There was a movie called *Less Than Zero* in the eighties. There's something about it that always resonated with me—being surrounded by rich kids, surrounded by people, but never feeling like you belong, like you're utterly alone. Like when you're at the party but not at the party.

That's how I felt in those childhood years.

My mother tried. I remember feeling comforted when she hugged me, but she worked often on the swing shift or afternoon shift. It felt like she was always working, and when she was home, she was exhausted and only wanted to sit and watch TV.

When she was off from work, she would take me to do fun things. We'd go to Niagara Falls, Clifton Hill, the Rainbow Mall, or for Chinese food. She kissed my booboos. She made me feel better when I felt down. But she didn't know how to take the darkness away.

"What's wrong?" she would say.

"I don't know," I would snip back.

I didn't know how to express the feeling of less than zero. No sparkle. Unwanted. Alone.

I didn't process the feelings I had when I found out my birth certificate had no father. And I didn't process the feelings I had when my mom told me about my dad at age twenty-one. It was like I disassociated from my body. I just listened, and I kept cutting cherries.

I left that day and went back to college. I remember feeling somewhat excited to know the truth.

If it was rape, what does that say about me? Am I half bad? Am I evil? Thoughts raced through my mind.

I remember feeling betrayed by my mom's friends who took her to Toronto.

How come they never told me? How could they have left my mom? Or let him take her? Do they know? Is this why I have such a big sex drive? Because my father is a rapist? Maybe my father was a sex freak rapist.

I thought back to those questions I had been seeking answers to. What did he look like? What kind of person was he? Now I knew. A rapist. A cheater, probably. The way I compartmentalized this when I was twenty-one was to stuff it way down and dismiss it.

Oh well, I'll never know him. I'm not bad. I know the story now. What else will I do with it?

Nothing. Put it away. Ignore it.

And so I did. I put it away, and I piled up a stack of bricks to build the walls of my labyrinth.

CHAPTER 2

All Too Serious

If you can't do something right, don't do it at all.

−JOAN CRAWFORD

I didn't know my great-grandparents, but my mother used to tell me she hated going to their house.

My grandmother's father owned an automobile dealership and repair garage called Schmitt's (my grandmother's maiden name). They originally sold and repaired Chrysler vehicles, then moved on to Volkswagen and Audi, and finally sold the business in 2017. Many of her brothers and sisters worked at and later owned and operated the garage. One of my uncles worked there his entire life.

Because my grandmother was one of the original children, we would get a ham, a box of chocolate, and a box of Franzia for Christmas every year from the dealership/garage. We always joked, saying, "That garage ham was really good."

My great-grandparents' house was right next to the dealership. My mother always described the house as a mansion, saying that the sitting room was so large that it housed the band and dance floor for her parents' wedding. The hand-carved molding was so impressive and ornate that they took the effort to save it to sell when the house was torn down.

When my mom and all her siblings visited the home as children, they had to sit perfectly still in a straight line on the couch without touching anything. They weren't allowed to run around and play. They were forced to wear stuffy, itchy clothes that they had to keep perfectly clean.

Clean and quiet. Quiet and clean.

My grandmother and great-aunts had been affected by their upbringing, and neurotic cleanliness was passed down in our family, like some families pass down alcoholism or high blood pressure. My grandmother was not of good mental capacity for most of my childhood, but occasionally, in her more lucid moments, she would clean. She would sanitize the brushes in the sink with alcohol and scrub the kitchen floor with two buckets and Comet cleaner. It made me think of the movie *Mommy Dearest*.

My mother picked up on this perfectionism and seriousness. It manifested in an OCD-like need to have an obsessively tidy apartment and a perfectly clean car. Every speck of dirt was picked up by hand if need be.

These habits were passed onto me like law. I had china dolls I could not play with, and my toys had to be kept organized and out of sight in the basement. That way I could play down there so the living room could always be tidy and neat.

When I would play outside with the neighbors and my knees would get dirty, my mom or grandma would yell at me and aggressively scrub them clean in the bathtub.

"Why are your knees *so* dirty, Joyel? What were you doing? How come this happens every day?!"

The message I received was that I was wrong for being me. I was a horrible child for playing and having fun. We have to be serious here. Look perfect and professional at age seven, eight, nine. Do all the things perfectly.

I once said, "Yes, Mommy Dearest," and I can tell you I *never* said that again.

Later in life, I learned about generational trauma being passed down, clearly evident in Jewish people, black and brown people, and other diversities. Still, I'd never noticed the trauma that my mother and grandparents may have been passing to me. It dawned on me—could this be generational trauma passed down from who-knows-how-long ago?

This environment made my mom into a hover mother, as she learned from my grandmother. She commented on what coat I wore based on the temperature outside, how I cooked, and what order of operations I followed, and was quick to say things like, "You're dressed like a slob." She oversaw how I cut the cake and took out the garbage, micromanaging me to ensure the knot was tight and the hole was closed.

I absorbed this seriousness and can see it in the photos of me as early as age four. My face was mostly stoic, whether I was jumping in the pool, trying my mom's shoes on, or emptying her purse. No smiling, no joy. I was busy, focused. Just like my grandmother doing the dishes.

When I was little, and someone was taking a photo of me, I imagine I would think, *What are you taking a picture of me for?* I'd be annoyed at the interruption.

And so, there was no lightheartedness in my home on an everyday basis.

Of course, there was festivity during the holidays when the booze flowed and different people were around. But most days it was quiet, stern, and serious. No fun. It was all business, function, survival, moving on from this task to the next, hardworking.

It was all too serious.

It's interesting that even though my mother and I essentially grew up in similar environments, we coped differently. My mother hated being criticized and thus always tried to be perfect. She became a very compliant person as a way of staying off my grandmother's radar. I, on the other hand, was defiant. The hover mother did not fare well with me, and my reaction to it turned me into a fiercely independent person, which caused a lot of strife between us. I wanted no hovering. I wanted to be free.

I have a palpable resentment of the seriousness built in me from all this control. I often feel like Sarah in *Labyrinth* shouting, "It's not fair!" to her father and stepmother. It doesn't feel fair that my childhood created these thick walls in the maze I've been painfully knocking into for decades.

The fun in my life became food, alcohol, adventure, adrenaline, and the next challenge. I was always looking outside of myself for an antidote to the heaviness I felt inside. I still struggle with knowing how to rest and how to let go of perfection. It's a puzzle in the labyrinth that I have yet to solve completely.

One step at a time.

CHAPTER 3

The Lawn

We've begun to raise daughters more like sons...
but few have the courage to raise our sons more like our daughters.

–GLORIA STEINEM

"You're always taking things the wrong way."

It was a refrain I heard often from my mother during childhood. The women in my family must have told me at least a thousand times that I was too sensitive. I would cry as my knees were getting scrubbed or when I didn't want to wear the dress, and they'd chastise me for my emotions.

In contrast, my grandpa had hardly any say or input in what I did. And so, I gravitated to spending more time with him. While the women were telling me I was wrong in the feelings that I did have, my grandpa was the way out.

He would let me weed the garden with him or stand over his shoulder while he was working on something on his workbench. He would ride bikes with me. He would praise things done well. He quizzed me on my spelling and gave me money for a good report card. He went to my softball games and my rifle matches. When I was little, he put me on his bike in a baby carriage, and when I got older, he taught me how to ride my first bike. It was a black bike intended for boys, likely a hand-me-down from my cousin. He let me climb trees. He didn't mind my dirty knees, not one bit.

But he was quiet, didn't talk much, and always had that serious face on him. I used to worry about his stern face, thinking he was upset.

"What's wrong?" I'd ask.

"Nothing, why?"

"You look mad."

"I'm not. I'm just serious."

He thought deeply about the next task, the next to-do on the list.

My uncle Buddy once told me that he had never heard the words "I love you" from my grandpa until he was over forty years old. He may have been quiet and stern, but I always felt accepted for who I was.

Once, when I was seven years old, I wanted to mow the lawn, so I asked Grandpa.

"No," he said, "girls can't do that, and you're too little."

I thought, *Oh yeah? Watch me!*

I proceeded to go out to the shed, lug the push lawn mower out, and try to pull-start it. I was too little and couldn't get the engine to turn over. Grandpa came out and started it for me.

"Make sure you go in a straight line," he said. "See where that wheel mark is? The next time you come down that row, make sure the other wheel is right on top of it so you don't miss any of the grass."

I remember feeling so excited. I push-mowed our third-of-an-acre yard. I felt proud, like I proved myself to my grandpa that day. It was my first memory of having to prove myself as a female, that I could do something as well as a man, and it wouldn't be the last.

I still like mowing the lawn.

Grandpa realized who I was and how I operated. When he noticed that I was watching too much TV, instead of criticizing me, he cut out a clipping from a newspaper about a kid who hadn't watched any TV for a year.

"I bet you can't do that."

"Sure I can," I insisted. All seriousness, all grit.

"I will bet you a hundred dollars you can't last a whole year."

I went a whole year without TV except for walking by when it was on in the house or the rare occasion of seeing a movie with my friends.

I grabbed onto this passionate persistence. It was a tool I'd use over and over again.

But I didn't realize that while it served me at work, it would not serve me in life and overall happiness. I focus almost to a fault. I can be blunt to the point that it's taken out of context as assertive and rude. I can notice these traits in others and point them out. I am sensitive to them.

More bricks in the labyrinth walls I was laying.

All too serious, all too focused.

CHAPTER 4

Just a Minute!

Where there is no struggle, there is no strength.

−OPRAH

When I was maybe four years old, my world was my playroom in my grand-parents' basement. I would spend hours arranging my Barbie village, playing with the dollhouse my grandpa built, and constructing cities, shops, and restaurants for Barbie. I'd whiz around on my Strawberry Shortcake roller skates, swirling around the support poles so fast. Or I'd hang from the open stairs like they were monkey bars.

The basement was my playground. Aside from needing a snack or a drink, I could tuck away and entertain myself. It was my safe space where I was insulated from my grandmother's episodes.

Back then everyone assumed my grandmother was manic depressive, but now, based on conversations my mom and I have had with doctors about her symptoms, we think her diagnosis would be psychotic. She would hallu-cinate or be completely delusional. She would talk to the walls like you were not there. No one knows the root cause of this, but my grandmother and all her sisters, except for Aunt Frannie, all had some form of mental illness that flared up when their father passed away.

One day, when I was little, I got busy playing downstairs and didn't realize how badly I had to use the restroom. The bathroom was right across the hall from the basement door upstairs, and I remember thinking what a good thing it was that it was so close.

I ran up the open staircase in the middle of the tiny house wearing my navy blue corduroy button-down pants. I despised the thick material. They limited my movement, and I detested the color. But mostly, I *hated* the buttons.

I stood in the bathroom trying to get the stupid buttons undone with my sweaty little hands, but I couldn't do it. As I urgently fumbled, I realized I needed help fast. I ran around the corner into the kitchen, where Grandma stood doing dishes.

I remember thinking, *She's dressed today.*

She had on an apron and everything. This was a rare occasion, and it became more so as her mental health deteriorated. But that day, she almost looked like a typical grandparent, the kind who would smile warmly at a wiggly four-year-old who was doing her best to squirm out of her blue, button-down corduroys.

But looks can be deceiving.

Back in the day, shock therapy was the treatment for the type of mental health issues Grandma and her siblings had. Many of them suffered greatly from the treatments, and because of this, my grandfather never pressured my grandmother into treatment. I was close to one of my great-aunts, but I never knew what she was like before the shocks. The entire time I'd known her, she was introverted and barely spoke, almost mute. When she did speak, it was so soft you could barely hear her.

Two of my grandmother's sisters, Eleanor and Francis (Aunt Ellie and Aunt Frannie), lived together and never married. Francis was very much of sound mind, but I assume she felt she needed to care for Eleanor.

Aunt Frannie and Ellie became staples in my life. They were so very kind and frequently babysat me. Every time I visited, they had fun things to do at their house. We made pencil holders with glue, napkins, glitter, and frosting containers. We colored, played games, baked cookies, made Barbie clothes with fancy napkins, painted our nails, and played with their mini tea set. They took me shopping, out to eat, and to the movies. They bought me my first swimming pool. My great-aunts spoiled me, and my cousins never failed to tell me so.

It's okay; they were right.

While my great-aunts were a bright spot in my childhood, my grandmother was not. Her mental health, personal care, and hygiene began to decline the older I got.

I remember that she would magically perk up when the social security check arrived. She would put on her coat and wait for my grandpa to come home to go shopping, and I would get dragged with them. We always went up Transit Road to Twin Fair or K-Mart. As I got older, I realized it was a travesty to be seen in a K-Mart, but at a young age, I didn't care. I would poke around the toy section and look at the Barbies and model airplanes. I wanted them both. Swimming pools and bikes. I wanted it all.

Grandma eventually stopped all cooking and cleaning the house by herself. My mom picked up the cooking, and my grandpa picked up most of the cleaning. My grandmother would go days without showering. On an up day, she would get out the good china and set the dining room table.

I would excitedly ask, "Who is coming to dinner, Grandma?"

She would say, "The boogie man!" and laugh.

I would turn around and run, afraid not of the boogie man but of her.

I remember once trying to clip her toenails when she was sleeping because they grossed me out. They were thick and curled. She moved, and I got too scared and gave up.

Because of my grandmother, I never wanted to have anyone over. It wasn't until I was much older that I had that one friend I trusted not to think I was a horrible person for having a crazy grandmother. Her name was Ann Clare. Ann was over and hugged my grandmother once, and I thought that was so strange.

Why are you touching her? I thought. *Ew. Stay away.*

If I summoned the courage to have other friends over, I typically warned them and then didn't introduce her to them.

"That's my crazy grandmother. Just ignore her," I'd say.

So you can see how, at four years old, squirming in my corduroys on that particular day, I thought it was unusual that she was up, dressed, and wearing an apron. She was cooking and busy and focused on those dishes, and I thought, maybe, just maybe, she'd be normal for once.

"Grandma, help me; I have to pee!" I said

"JUST A MINUTE!!" she shouted.

Our house was tiny, and the bathroom was next to the kitchen. I kept running in and out and screaming for help. And she just kept shouting back at me in her nasty yell-at-you voice.

"Help, Grandma, I can't get my pants unbuckled!" My little heart thumped, and my bladder throbbed.

"JUST A MINUTE!!"

Finally, the warm pee ran down my corduroy legs, and I started to cry. I was standing against the wall in the bathroom. She finally came around the corner, and I stood frozen in fear and shame. She promptly turned me around and spanked me. It was the only time I remember being spanked.

I was furious at the injustice.

Why am I getting spanked? I thought. *Pee is a bodily function.*

Of course, I wouldn't say I liked that she was delusional, talked to walls, chain-smoked, didn't get dressed most days, and came out of the bathroom after the occasional shower butt-naked, but those things didn't affect me like this. This was personal. I was mad. It was the turning point when all my feelings toward my grandmother turned to hate.

Bridge burned. Betrayal.

That one traumatic moment placed cinder blocks that would form the wall of distrust of all people. Don't ask for help. Don't trust women. For sure, never trust your grandmother.

It's funny how such a simple incident can make you hold onto pain for such a long time. I never spoke to her or my mother about it. I buried the hate deep down like a walnut I swallowed that would never get digested and stay in my side.

CHAPTER 5

Stargazer

*Astronomy compels the soul to look upwards and leads
us from this world to another.*

–PLATO

Even amidst the identity crisis of who I was, who my dad was, and how I fit
in my household, something else was blossoming that pointed me straight
to who I would become. There were flickers of hope and light. There were
sparks of joy and people whose paths crossed mine and planted seeds of a
future brighter than I could have imagined. Just like a spark plug and igni-
tion exciter are needed to spark and light the engine, I can see how these
people purposefully came into my life.

Jamie and Jackie lived across the street, but I had never met them because they went to public school instead of Catholic school. One day, when
I was maybe five or six years old, I asked my mom if I could go across the
street and play with those girls.

"Sure," she shrugged.

"What do I say?"

She coached me to knock on the door and ask if the girls could play. I
remember her watching me cross the street to make sure I made it safely. I

nervously walked up to the house and knocked.

When the door swung open, I said, "Um… there is a little girl who lives here, or two…umm…do you think they could come out and play?"

Mrs. P smiled and said, "Jackie is out back on the swing set. You can go out there. Jamie is at school. She's in second grade."

I edged around the house and saw Jackie swinging. I steeled my nerves. "Do you want to play?" I asked.

"Sure. You can swing." She pointed to the second swing next to her. "I'm in kindergarten," Jackie informed me. "I skipped school today." I asked her if she was sick and she said "No, I just didn't feel like going."

I remember thinking, *What?* I'm a big rule follower, so it seemed unbelievable to me that she would be skipping school just because she felt like it.

Soon after, Jamie came home on the bus, and she remembers I brought some robot toy over, which I have no recollection of now.

The three of us had so much fun growing up. We played hide and seek, ghost in the graveyard, tag, freeze tag, and cartoon freeze tag. Jamie and Jackie had a pool, and we swam in it frequently. We played school inside their house when the weather wasn't great, and we played baseball in their backyard when it was. We colored and played board games. Christmas morning, we'd run over and show each other our presents. When their dad built a new fireplace in the den, we used the loose bricks to make our Barbies a cool restaurant.

We never ran out of things to do together. Jackie was obsessed with Troll dolls, and her room was full of them. I remember that, in summer, we left an epically long Monopoly game up in their garage. We rode bikes with the other neighbor kids, too. We weren't supposed to go into the burnt-down house on the corner, but we did. We ventured into the backfield and found a swampy spot that would freeze over in the winter, and we'd ice skate. One time, they came over to my house to play in the backyard on a warm summer day, and when it started to pour down rain, we made a muddy, grassy slip-and-slide. We just kept running and sliding. It was the BEST.

The neighborhood kids allowed me to be me. The had fun imaginations and made me realize how much play is and was an essential part of myself. I am grateful for them and hold a special place in my heart, although I never realized it then. It took me a long time to find that girl who knows how to play and allow her to come back out.

Jamie and Jackie's dad was into the lunar and solar eclipses and would host watch parties. He'd set out lay-down lawn chairs, drinks, snacks, and blankets, and we'd stare at the sky. He taught us how to spot the mid-August shooting stars when the Earth passes through the Swift-Tuttle comet tail in the Perseid meteor shower. The slowness of watching it all unfold never bothered me.

I'd leave those parties asking life's big questions.

Where do we come from? How big is the Universe?

Questions of wonder and science began, and I'd go home and look up articles in our Britannica Encyclopedia set that lived in my room. I'd take books out of the library and subscribe to science magazines. I imagined becoming an astrophysicist or an engineer. I just knew I liked looking at the stars.

To this day, in mid- to late August, I climb in a sleeping bag on the deck with my kiddos and look for the shooting stars. Something about looking up into that dark night sky takes your breath away. Looking at the sky makes me feel a part of something greater than myself. It makes my mistakes and worries seem silly.

Some people have a fear of looking into the vast sky. It's overwhelming thinking about the size of the Universe; I get it. But for me, it's exciting and peaceful at the same time. It's calming and beautiful. Like being awed by a rainbow, I am captivated by the night sky. The moon, the clouds, a sunset, a sunrise, the beach, a field of corn. I frequently bike in the rolling hills of Upstate New York and think, "in God's country," despite my issues with the word God. Appreciation for it all is like giving thanks to God for all that is. In those moments, I feel the walls I've built shudder and crumble.

I'm not sure how or when, but we all grew apart. I remember when I went to public high school, I would ride the bus. Jackie was a year older and said I could only sit with her for the first day. She was dressed in goth and wasn't very popular. She was quiet and kept to herself. Our paths rarely crossed in high school, and sometimes, I feel sad we never kept that friend-ship up. We had so many good childhood memories. The fun, adventure, and stargazing created a sense of magic and joy in my life, and I've found those same themes of fun and following joy in my life now.

I had forgotten.

And I wouldn't remember until years later when Lacy reminded me.

Firefly

I am the Firefly
I am Sam
Give Happiness
I wonder, are all the Fireflies
Fairies
Are they all so magical
In my backyard
Camping in Cooperstown
Flying over the creek
I am the Firefly
Special and a sign of hope
A flicker in the darkness
A flicker as a pointer
If love is light, and I am love, and I am light, how do we see the light
    without the dark
How do we know how sweet the rest is without the work
How do we know how special the Firefly is if it were not for the
    darkness it has flown through
How do we know how sweet the fruit is if we have only sugar to
    compare

CHAPTER 6

Annie Banana

Today you are you! That is truer than true!
There is no one alive who is you-er than you!

—DR. SEUSS

Ann was my first friend at my Catholic grammar school. I would call her Annie Banana, and she would roll her eyes and dramatically sigh even though she knew it was a term of endearment. We rode the same bus, and I remember yelling out to her that first day she got on.

"Ann, sit with me!"

Another girl, Lynn, did the same. "Ann, sit with *me*!"

Ann looked at us and politely said, "How about we take turns. I'll sit with you today and Joyel tomorrow...we'll alternate"

I got the feeling she didn't really want to sit with me, but I didn't care. I thought to myself, *She is so nice and very fair.*

Ann and Lynn were in the first reading group in first grade, meaning they were reading at a third-grade, big-chapter-book level. I was like, *Whoa —she is so smart.* I would go over to Ann's house, and she would read Dr. Seuss so fast with a funny, silly voice, and I remember thinking, *She is nice, smart, and fun.*

PART 1 | BUILDING THE WALLS

I was in the third reading group in first grade—the lowest. I don't remember reading much at home, if at all.

When I was at Ann's house, her mom was in teaching mode almost all the time, and I could see how and why Ann was so smart. She had been in an environment where her mom was actively engaged in her learning and development and frequently turned those learnings into fun games. Even at such a young age, I noticed and cataloged that my house was different.

At school, I felt frustrated waiting for all the slow kids and was shocked and annoyed that I was in this group with what I thought were a bunch of dummies. Eventually, our teacher, Mrs. Shaun, moved me up to the middle reading group, and I remember feeling so proud and happy the day she told me.

At that age, the boys were into coloring or driving their Matchbox cars up and down the long tables, and I remember longing to do what they did. It seemed like so much more fun, but I stuck with the girls.

Not for long.

I loved Mrs. Shaun. She was kind and warm. We were lucky enough to have her move from kindergarten to first grade with us, and I was so happy when they told us. There were so many cool toys to play with in the rooms.

I remember loving nap time in kindergarten. After recess, we would come in and take our mat, which was basically a floor mat that you'd put in front of your kitchen counter. We could put the mat anywhere we wanted in the room. I always thought that was the best part. It was fun to sleep in a new and different place each time.

One time, I put my mat under the tables where we sat. This day, Mrs. Shaun sat down at this table, and I rolled over and suddenly could see right up her skirt. It just looked dark and didn't seem too interesting, but I couldn't turn away.

I knew looking was wrong, and guilt flooded my little body. I felt like I was evil. It's the first time I remember feeling shame. I never told anyone, not even in my first confession, but it was something I wrestled with as a young six- or seven-year-old.

Second grade was not so much fun. The teacher was mean, and my hair was always stuck in the chairs and the scooters. Our school "gym" was in the basement and wasn't big or tall enough to play real games. So they used Fisher Price basketball nets, and we rolled around on these friggin' scooters all the time playing scooter basketball or scooter hockey. I hated those things.

Somewhere in second grade, fear and depression began to sink in, and I had no idea where they were coming from. I was afraid of everyone—my teacher, Father Bone, my grandmother, God, my mom. I got yelled at for what seemed to be all the time, especially for not remembering to bring my pants home. We wore uniforms to school, which included a pleated blue and white plaid skirt, and in the winter, we wore pants under the skirt during outside recess.

"If you wore the pants to school *and* at recess, why can't you remember to bring them HOME?" My mom would scream at me from the top of the stairs after shouting my whole name.

I constantly felt that feeling of not belonging, shame, and doing everything wrong. My body was putting on weight, and I was uncomfortable. I remember feeling that I didn't fit in with my family and that maybe I wasn't wanted. My one and only friend wasn't my friend; she was just nice and fair. I felt like all the kids at school thought I was dumb and fat.

This was the age I noticed my skin was darker than my family's. It was the age when I realized that I didn't have a dad, and I questioned my mother about my father. It was the age when that big blank spot on my birth certificate became a gaping hole in my heart.

Ann's friendship and her fun, lighthearted family became an escape. I would eat dinner there and listen to her brother compliment her mom's food.

"How do you make this chicken so good?" he'd fawn.

I would listen to her dad pretend the cob of corn was a typewriter and make a ding sound after he ate every row. I would bask in her sister's cool new wave music. We would spend hours in her basement playing board games, and I'd run to the other side of the room where her dad was putting together model airplanes. He would talk endlessly about them, and I'd quietly listen, not knowing then what a huge role those planes would play in my life years later.

We'd laugh at her dad's funny expressions. "Norm, how are we going to get up that cherry tree?!"

Her family would talk and make fun of farting noises. In my house, we didn't fart, or if we did, you just ignored it. They all seemed like a fun bunch of crazy bananas. Ann and her family were and are still so charismatic. They bring light and lighthearted play and fun to all situations.

She and I also bonded over the type of house we had. We lived in the more modest homes in the area and sometimes got teased for it on the bus. She would tell me when she got made fun of, and I remember wanting to go beat up those boys for her. Even though our families didn't have much money, she had a swimming pool, which I loved and she could care less about. I was always trying to get her to go swimming.

It's interesting how the fun of childhood so seamlessly weaves with the heartache. Even though I know I was hurting at this time, my mind swims with memory after memory of the little delights of being with Ann, like all the hours spent playing outside in her backyard. Her dad made a treehouse, and we'd climb up there and pass the time playing pretend. We'd adventure together like brave explorers to the far back of the woods. Her dad even let me try to drive the lawn mower once (and only once), and I ran it into a bush.

She invented the word "ERR," which we used as an adjective for anything cute—like an old man or a squishy stuffed animal. Even at my thirtieth high school reunion, someone said, "Remember you and Ann used to use that word ERR all the time?"

Ann came to my house occasionally and accepted my grandmother and my quiet, stern household. We ate fireballs on the living room floor while we watched *Labyrinth* and many other shows. My mom would take us to fun places when she wasn't working. And even though we barely had any classes together in high school, we would call each other after school every day.

Ann was my very best friend, the person who probably knew me best, and still, she had no idea how deep and dark the labyrinth really was. She had no idea the pain that was brewing in my heart all those years.

CHAPTER 7

Escape Artist

Es-ca-pe. I wonder what that means. It's funny.
It's spelled just like the word escape.

–DORY, *FINDING NEMO*

My love for playing outside alone started in elementary school. I would go into the woods, jump on the rocks in the creek, and follow the tree line to the Ransom Oaks housing development. Or I'd walk in the fields across the street behind Jamie and Jackie's house to North French Road. It was only about a quarter of a mile, but to my second-grade self, it was a long way. Now, this area is all developments with sparkly new homes.

One crisp fall afternoon, I played outside in the woods, climbed trees, and swung from branches. I was a few houses down, and when I started to walk home, I noticed the sudden urge to poop. We were not a camping or hiking family, so I had no idea what to do. I looked around and thought, *Should I run back in the woods?* I didn't think I could make it that far, but I couldn't make it to the house either.

I decided that behind our shed in the far back of my yard was where it would happen. I pulled down my pants and pooped behind there at the edge of our property. I thought for sure my grandpa would find out and yell at me or that the neighbors saw and would rat me out. I felt deep shame, and I carried it around with me. I didn't realize how heavy a burden it was until it was time to make my first confession.

Like all good Catholic kids, I had to make my first confession and first holy communion. The teachers and nuns told me to think about things I felt bad about. They instructed us to think about the Ten Commandments and any times we broke them, like lying or disobeying our parents.

I couldn't think of anything but going to the bathroom outside and looking up Mrs. Shaun's skirt, so I made up other more plausible, less terrible confessions. I thought that pooping in the backyard was worse than disobeying your mom. So I confessed to sins I'd heard but were not true. I decided to carry my evilness around with me instead. In my young mind, God already knew I was evil, so what difference did it make?

I also didn't confess to thinking about kissing boys in church. It's not like they were my neighbors' spouses or something, so what was the big deal? But the self-justification didn't work. I knew it must be bad and wrong and that I should feel guilty about it.

I wasn't swearing then, but essentially I was like, *Forget that shit.* I despised the white-bearded, wizard-looking guy in the sky knowing every damn thing I did. And I hated feeling bad for pooping in the backyard. Screw that guy. I was so angry about learning how to shame myself for every wrongdoing, every selfish act, every forgetful mistake that I decided that both this religion thing and the house I lived in were not for me.

Somewhere along the way, I got the idea to run away. And so I started to plan. At this time, my mom worked the swing shift at the Amherst Police Department, and I waited for her to go to work at eleven that night. I was in bed but fully dressed under the covers. I had my Garfield suitcase packed and ready under my bed.

When the time came, I got out of bed, pulled out my suitcase, and started down the stairs. I can remember the adrenaline. My plan was to live in the woods right next to school, brush my teeth in the school bathroom, and still go straight to school each morning. I figured education was important and that if I was going to school, too, no one would notice I was missing. No cops would be called.

As I was about to sneak out, my aunt, who was living with us at the time, caught me. The stupid creaky stairs tipped her off.

"What do you think you're doing?" she demanded.

I pressed my shoulders back and straightened my spine. "I'm leaving," I announced.

"Nah, why don't you go back to bed and think about this."

And somehow, she convinced me to stay. I begrudgingly agreed and went to bed. There was always tomorrow.

I wonder what the conversation between her and my mom had been the next day. Maybe she never told her. Neither of them ever brought it up to me.

In reality, I knew there wasn't going to be a tomorrow. I knew I wasn't going to go. But I still remember dreaming of it, just like Dorothy in *The Wizard of Oz*. I was obsessed with that movie.

I think I watched it for the first time at my mom's best friend's mother's house. I called her Grandma K. I had a real relationship with this woman, far more than my own grandmother. My mom and her best friend had grown up together, and her siblings were like a part of our family. I called them aunts and uncles, and their kids were my cousins.

Grandma K always called me a Latin beauty. She was just about the only person who ever told me I was beautiful. Around her, I felt like I was allowed to sparkle, like there was a part of me that actually did sparkle.

We were at Grandma K's for a holiday, and my cousins and I were watching *The Wizard of Oz*. I was mesmerized. I couldn't stop thinking about it. I could easily relate to Dorothy's wish to be somewhere else and to her always feeling unwanted and alone. And, of course, I related to wanting to run away.

Running away became a constant theme for me.

Escape by compulsively overeating, drinking, consuming TV, social media, working out, adventure. Escape the current stress or the next. Escape the feelings. Find the nearest exit. Wish to be somewhere else, anywhere else, somewhere over the rainbow.

But I couldn't. I was stuck wandering around a never-ending maze of the same repeating issues. I would always be the fatherless brown girl trapped in a fat body. No matter where I ran, there I was.

'Ello

'Ello Love
you Latin beauty
you fish
you miracle worker
you magic bringer
Your beautiful face
Here, play with my jewels and white party dress gloves
Roller-skate in the basement
Bike the trail
Do all the things, my love, all the things.

CHAPTER 8

Fat Fall

I told you
That we could fly
'Cause we all have wings
But some of us don't know why

–INXS

"Hey, Joyel, why are you *so fat*?"

I'm fat? I thought to myself.

The ribbed rubber floor of the bus was all I could look at as my world came crashing down.

The mean boys in the back of the bus yelled it for everyone to hear, but I'd hear it screamed a thousand more times throughout the world. Teachers, family, people shouting out of the car windows when I walked or biked down the street, men in parking lots, mean girls in college. It reverberated throughout my life because I let it. Because I believed it.

"Hey, fatso, don't sit on me."

I walked up the bus aisle, finding a seat as quickly as possible. The taunting seemed to go on for hours. I learned to sit up front, but that didn't stop them. I lowered my head and looked out the window, tears running down my face.

Once, on the bus during the bullying, a friend from Girl Scouts, Sally, wanted to console me and didn't know how or what to say.

"Hey, Joyel…"

"What?" I snapped at her.

I was convinced Sally was going to make fun of me, too.

Caught off guard, she said, "Um… ah… you know you're my friend, right?"

I smiled, and we both laughed. At that moment, I appreciated her, and I think (or hope) I said thanks. Her kindness felt like a tiny flicker in the darkness.

As an adult trying to make sense of the past, I looked back at old photos of my childhood self around the time the bullying started. My hair was chopped between second and third grades, and it turned me into a frizzy, curly mess. I'd also put on weight at that time, but it wasn't apparent to me then. I was a wild, fun kid who didn't notice her body until it was noticed for her, and not kindly.

The bus wasn't the only taunting; it was just the beginning. It seemed to be pervasive from then on out. From that point forward, every time anyone teased me about anything, I assumed it was negative and about my weight, even if it was by my sweet Great-Aunts Frannie or Ellie.

When my aunt made fun of me for getting a bra at such a young age, I got upset. Taunting. I would get accused of being oversensitive or yelled at by my mom for overreacting. Every mean comment anyone ever said, every dirty look, every awkwardness, I thought it must be about my weight.

Riding bikes on Dodge Road, people would yell out of their cars, "Hey, fatso, your tire is flat."

Walking into work at Tops grocery store when I was sixteen, someone hung out of the window of their car screaming at me, "Hey, fat ass!"

In freshman year of college, a girl from New York City, whom I had been hanging around with in a group of friends, called me into her dorm room to talk to me and told me, "I can't be friends with fat people."

Even at Ann's house, I'd watch carefully how many chips she ate, and I would only eat the same amount. But when I ate the whole veggie tray, her mom was aghast. She ranted over and over how she couldn't believe I ate the entire thing.

Throughout my youth, seemingly every adult I ever met commented on how I was getting chunky and how I should try to lose it now. The heaviness of the shame was a thousand times the heaviness on my bones.

I also carried deep shame for something I didn't even know I did. Shame for being who I was. I felt like I was inherently bad.

At this same age, third grade, I went to the doctor, and he put me and my mom on a 1,000-calorie diet. I can still remember the paper on the bulletin board in the kitchen listing the foods, serving sizes, and calories. Only eat these foods, it said, and it was broken up into dairy, starch, fruit and vegetables, meat, and fat. I remember eating the celery and cottage cheese, the Bison blueberry yogurt, the rice cakes, and plain tuna.

Soon after, my mom took me to a different doctor, and he felt me up right in front of her.

I looked at her like, *What the heck?*

He verbally explained that he could tell if this was simply baby fat or a real problem by the amount of fat around my vagina. The expression on my mom's face validated my concern.

This doesn't seem right, I thought.

We basically ran out of there, never returned, and, of course, never spoke about it.

Don't look at it. Don't talk about it.

We eventually made our way to Weight Watchers. All the women were welcoming and praised me for showing up. I was the only child in that fluorescent-lit room with the large, white, stick-on-tiled floor in the business office on Sheridan Drive. I hadn't even reached double digits in age yet, and here I was in a room full of grown women talking about being overweight and stepping on the scale in front of everyone. Before high school, I had been to Weight Watchers four times.

As an adult, I did many other diets. Pretty much every diet you can think of. Fasting, juicing, cabbage soup, rainbow, Atkins, keto, paleo, multiple different diet pills from the doctor, diet pills off the shelf, Body for Life with Oprah, Biggest Loser and Jillian Michaels books, Beachbody, South Beach diet, the Zone diet, Overeaters Anonymous, food addicts, Geneen Roth eating guidelines, bodybuilders diets, Weight Watchers about a million times, clean eating magazine diets, Michael Pollan's book diet, Kripalu integrative weight loss diet. This goes on and on.

During this lifelong exploration of my food history, I had to determine when I started overeating and why. It was about the same time, third grade.

My grandmother had made fresh brownies with walnuts on top. They sat in the kitchen in the corner of our white countertop near the refrigerator. That's where the sweets always went. Kuchen, Entenmann's, cookies. My grandmother had a sweet tooth. On this day, she made brownies. I was watching something on TV and ran back and forth from the living room to the kitchen, grabbing a brownie and re-arranging the plate to make it look like I hadn't taken any. By the fourth or fifth brownie, making it look the same was hard, but I took it anyway. Sugar was my first drug of choice.

Sister Sheila was the principal the entire time I was at my Catholic grammar school (kindergarten through eighth grade). Like many nuns, she was somber, serious, quiet, but had a mean streak. A bit of a temper. She was a heavyset woman with salt and pepper gray bangs hanging neatly out of her head dressing. Her office was right in the middle of the school, with the upper grades to the left and the lower grades to the right. She could yell and snap into anger at the drop of a hat. You walked in straight lines. You didn't mess around. She scared me.

As students, we were commanded to show evidence of respect. For example, when she walked in the room, we were all supposed to stand up. She would inspect our uniforms and the classroom. I suspect she would also give the teacher a once over, but I was too nervous to really pay attention. She dealt with the problem children who spoke back to teachers, didn't listen, and were disruptive.

I never got sent down to Sister Sheila's office, but I did get called down. Mostly to talk about my weight. What was my new diet? How many calories? What did I bring for lunch? What plan was I going to follow?

I once had a rash on my arm and went to the school nurse. For some reason, she sent me to Sister Sheila's office. Sister Sheila told me that if I had a rash on my arm, I probably would have it on my stomach and legs, too. She made me stand in front of her and lift up my skirt and shirt. She touched my stomach, pinched it, and had a smiling smirk on her face that I wanted to punch.

I didn't like this one bit.

My mind raced. *Why wasn't the school nurse checking me? Why was I sent here? Why did she pinch my fat?*

I still think she just wanted to see how fat I was. Or maybe just point it out to me.

What was that smirk? Was she happy because I was fatter than her? My teenage mind tried to make sense of it all.

Being overweight herself, sometimes she would share her plan, her diet, and her workouts or call me down to ask how I was doing.

"I burned a hundred calories on the elliptical and had celery for dinner," she'd say.

I wanted to scream, *I don't freaking care!*

I never really knew what to say. I stood there awkwardly, playing with my skirt pleats, staring down, and answering her questions minimally. At that age, I ate what was given to me. I wasn't fixing my dinner. If my mom was on a diet, *we* were on a diet. If we weren't, we weren't. Either way, I felt like a failure.

I was always the only fat kid in the room. Even though there were a couple of other chubby boys, I was the only fat girl, and I felt a hundred times bigger than the biggest boys. I felt incredibly alone.

This time, I actually went home and told my mom. I told her that I didn't like Sister Sheila and didn't like it when she made me lift up my shirt. I felt violated. I felt sick.

My mother made it seem like I was too sensitive and overreacting and that it wasn't a big deal. For a long time, I blamed her for not advocating for me and not teaching me how to speak up respectfully. I felt betrayed by my mother. I felt like she was on Sister Sheila's side, and I hated her for that.

This was not the first or the last time my mother betrayed me. Several times, when I would tell her what, to me, were private and embarrassing facts, I would find out later that she had shared them, laughing at me with my aunt or her friends. My mom's closest friend would tell me or call me out on something, and I would know she had blabbed.

There's a part in the movie *Labyrinth* when Jareth, the Goblin King, gives Hoggle a piece of poisoned fruit to give to Sarah. Jareth wants to halt Sarah's progress through the winding maze, and he hopes to exploit the trust Hoggle has built with Sarah to trick her. It works. She falls for the betrayal. Sarah eats the fruit and falls into a dreamlike state that steals hours away from her mission.

Betrayal was a concept I learned early on. All women, even those closest to you, will betray you. You never know if they're on your side or carrying poisoned fruit meant to trick you.

CHAPTER 9

Everyone Hates You

Maybe you have to know the darkness before you can appreciate the light.

While I felt like a big fat loser because the boys and Sister Sheila told me so, I thought I could still count on my girlfriends.

Boy, was I wrong.

I think it's probably common to have a fear that everyone hates you, but to be directly told is quite another. Fourth-grade girls, in particular, can be fucking vicious.

Every day for lunch, we marched in a single file line down the concrete stairs that were polished to look like marble, our shoes gripping the black, adhesive, anti-slip strips, moving through the swinging doors into the tan, painted, cement floor basement of our cafeteria/gymnasium/auditorium/ dance hall. (I didn't realize how low the ceilings in that stairwell were until later in life when I went back and almost hit my head.) The entire school would pile into the cafeteria, which was just a bunch of long folding tables and chairs grouped in the basement to the right, passing the open space we used as a gym every other day on the left. We would eat at the lunch tables, watching the boys trade ho-hos for oatmeal cookies while I begrudgingly ate my celery.

Shortly after lunch, every day, we would file up the cement stairs at the back of the basement and out into the playground/parking lot. All the kids would run to the playground, the fast kids claiming the swings, the tee-ter-totter, the merry-go-round, and then the slides. Being too fat and slow, I never recall getting a swing. I was too fat to play on the teeter-totter with any of the kids, so I stayed away from the playground, occasionally playing on the merry-go-round or going down the metal, hot-as-hell slide too fast and landing hard on the ground.

I would play king of the mountain on the snow banks and win using my girth to shove other kids down. This was one of my first exhibits of strength and taught me my weight and my girth might have some benefit. I'd play jump rope and hopscotch with the girls. I remember sliding around on the ice in the parking lot, once falling on the ice and getting the wind knocked out of me. But sometimes, we'd have fun exploring the edges of the play-ground/forest before getting caught.

For who knows what reason, I was happy on this particular day about going outside. I engaged with my friends and asked what they wanted to do today.

"Hey, should we play jump rope or softball?" I said to everyone and no one at the same time.

As we were walking up the stairs, one girl turned around angrily, bent over at the waist, and screamed in my face like a rabid dog.

"Everyone hates you!"

Shocked, I looked down and slowly continued walking up the dark staircase. The blood fell out of my face. The ground dropped away from my feet. I felt faint.

I immediately went into denial and thought, *She's crazy.*

I started going around asking my so-called friends.

"I don't know what she's talking about," Ann reassured me.

I went up to another girl and another until I'd talked to all the girls. I got some shrugs and cold shoulders.

Uh oh, maybe this is true, I wondered.

I have no memory of what happened after that, but I know there was screaming and crying in the parking lot. My next memory is sitting in our fourth-grade teacher's room. She was a short, stocky, mean teacher who only cared about gossiping in the hall with the third-grade teacher. The memory sharpens for me when our teacher tried to get us to talk.

It was me and two other girls who had been screaming at each other in the parking lot. We were placed in her room separated as far apart as possible. The lights were off because they were always off during lunch, and I assumed they stayed off to keep us calm. There was plenty of natural daylight coming in.

The girl who told me that everyone hated me was crying, and she eventually apologized. Ultimately, she said I was too bossy and always trying to control what the group was doing. I was numb, my eyes were puffy, and I had nothing else to say. I was hated for my bossiness, and there was nothing else I could do.

I took this to mean that fundamentally, down to my core, I was wrong for being who I am. I unconsciously resolved to hate all women and hate myself. And I vowed to look for more proof that all women are backstabbing bitches. Cinder blocks and an entire section of the labyrinth were built that day. Do you remember the Bog of Eternal Stench in *Labyrinth*? Well, that day, the Bog of Eternal Bitch was constructed in my maze.

My subconscious wired itself to say, *Women. Fear them. Hate them. Never, ever, EVER trust them.*

It was a puzzle I didn't unlock until twenty years into my career.

This statement—Everyone hates you—has been pervasive throughout my life. It's a scar that gets picked open frequently.

If I didn't get invited to a wedding, *See? Everyone hates you.*

If I wasn't asked to camp with friends even though I mentioned we needed a spot to stay, *See? Everyone hates you.*

Someone didn't text me back, *See? Everyone hates you.*

Didn't get invited to coworkers' going away parties, *See? Everyone hates you.*

My stepson spends more time with my mom than me, *See? Everyone hates you.*

I didn't get the job, didn't get asked out for drinks, didn't get a "miss you too" from a friend who moved away when I said I missed them, didn't get the office with a door at work (while my back-fill, at the same level, a middle-aged white man DID get the office with a door, the corner office actually)...

See? Everyone. Hates. You.

Although Ann was still my best friend, and we spoke on the phone nearly daily, fear crept in when she started to get close to another girl in our class. This other girl was funnier and skinnier than me. Ann laughed at her jokes, even though I didn't think she was funny. She was unique, had beautiful handwriting, learned how to tease her hair to look like a headbanger, and became increasingly popular. I feared I was getting ousted. There was something about her that I didn't like or trust.

So I would bring these things up to Ann, and she would not comment or say anything. I thought we were on board and aligned that we didn't like her. This was when three-way calls were brand new, and this girl talked Ann into calling me up and getting me to talk about her. Well, this backfired on Ann.

Ann brought up the girl, and I said, "You know we both hate her."

A half-hour later, Ann called me crying and explaining that she was on the phone line when I said that.

"Oh," I muttered. I never have the right words to say when I'm in shock.

I felt betrayed by both Ann and this girl. I was pissed. I didn't feel bad for Ann. I felt like it served her right. And I was so pissed at the girl that I never spoke to her again. She was a sneaky bitch. Written off. Another cinder block in the wall. Trust no one. Not boys. Not parents. Not girls. Not teachers. I was starting to learn I needed to be fiercely independent.

These two events have made me very cautious about new friends and even more careful about my words. If someone wants to be my friend, they had better climb that cinder block wall I had put up first. If they fail, they better try again. They better be super nice, start the conversation, ask me to do stuff, and be overly friendly, but not too much to be annoying. If I try to be friends with someone and they can't or don't seem to want to, then I put an all-stop to the efforts and even unfollow them. Because obviously, they must hate me.

It's made me cold, stand-offish, almost to the point of being rude. I don't get close to people I know who constantly talk about other people behind their backs. I am cautious about who I choose to let in. And, I hope if I ever was inadvertently rude to people, they understand why now. I hope they know that people have really good reasons to do what they do.

We're all just wandering through our labyrinths trying to make sense of the dead ends.

PART 2

It's Not Fair

CHAPTER 10

Not Good Enough to Puke

Owning our own story can be hard but not nearly as difficult as spending our lives running from it.

–BRENE BROWN

There was an after-school special on NBC that featured the mom from the show *Family Ties*, Meredith Baxter, called "Kate's Secret." It was about bulimia nervosa. I was glued to the television, watching her stuff packages of cookies in her mouth and then go behind the grocery store to vomit it up. Ever since the boys on the bus told me so, I knew I was fat, and I wondered if this puking thing could help me out. It seemed like an excellent idea.

I spent many years of my life obsessed with food. I was culturally conditioned at a very young age. One time, my mom and I were visiting my aunt in Seattle, and she made all this weird food I'd never had, like lentils and curry. I asked her one night if we would ever have normal food.

"What's normal food?" she pressed.

"Burgers," I answered without hesitation. But then I immediately thought, *Oh, I shouldn't have answered that; those are fattening.*

I knew on my seventh birthday that burgers were apparently bad for you. I would get motivated to work out, and I'd go to the library, take out books with workout plans, and do them in my basement playroom. When Olivia Newton John's video of her in a leotard, tights, headband, and leg warmers came on MTV, I'd get dressed in my dance tights and jump around the living room with her or Richard Simmons.

I didn't ever talk to anyone about my insecurities. My mom always knew something was wrong, but when she questioned me, I felt like I might get lectured, so I kept it all inside.

"Why aren't you happy?" she'd say. "What's wrong?"

I didn't realize that it was all tied to my less-than-zero self-worth and that I felt bad about everything. Hated, ugly, can't trust the girls, can't trust the boys, can't trust the adults, can't get skinny with this working out thing.

What's wrong with me? I'd think over and over.

But maybe, just maybe, this puking thing was the answer.

I had been in Girl Scouts ever since I could remember. I started attending meetings at Dodge Road Elementary School with a bunch of girls from the public school. The meetings were big, and the leaders and events were fun. Later, Ann and a few girls from our Catholic school decided to create our own troop.

Of course, I sold tons of Girl Scout cookies. The pretty, colored boxes arrived and filled our tiny dining room. I could smell the cookies even through the wrapping. We had ordered some for ourselves, too, and I ate and ate and ate. One day, when my mom was at work, I decided to try them all. I had no idea how many I went through, but I landed on Samoas as my favorite. I proceeded to the bathroom, but I could not make myself throw up.

Panic.

I took a toothbrush, stuck it down my throat, and tried to make myself throw up. Still nothing. I felt disgusting, and my body felt like it was pulsing from the sugar.

What was I going to do? I couldn't even do this! What's wrong with me?

Several times in my life, I've eaten to the point of actually being sick, my body naturally ejecting the food from one end or the other. That year, and probably several other years, I ate cookies for the customers I sold to, and we had to go back to the troop and get more to cover for my overeating. It wasn't until I was much older that I realized there was a name for this—binge-eating disorder.

During this dark chapter of my life, I felt like a failure in everything I attempted, whether it was running to the swings, making friends, or even puking.

Failure.

CHAPTER 11

Just Look Up

Religion is for people who fear hell, spirituality is for people who have been there.

—DAVID BOWIE

When I was between nine and twelve years old, I was terrified of airplanes. I had an irrational fear that every airplane I heard was on its way to crashing directly into me. I was so convinced that I would scream, yell, and carry on like it was for sure happening—right into me, personally.

It was a strange, abnormal fear coming from who knows where. I would hear a plane coming and shamefully excuse myself to the bathroom to plug my ears until it disappeared. I remember being at least twelve years old because I had to go into the bathroom during my twelfth birthday to hunker down until one passed.

One day, when I was at the Eastern Hills Mall, which is very close to the airport, I had a full-fledged panic attack in the parking lot. When planes fly into that airport, they are very low, and my fear exploded to a new level. I was screaming in the mall parking lot, and my mom was trying to calm me down.

"Just look up," she said.

This. Coming from the woman who had raised me in the family that never looked at anything.

But I did it. I tilted my head back while still hollering, my arms braced overhead to protect myself, and I stared petrified at the airplane. Its jet engines boomed louder than I had ever heard at home, and it felt massive in the sky above me. And yet, it safely flew right past me.

It calmed me down to look, to see the airplane belly, engines, and landing gear. They were so close and so loud. I wanted to wait and watch another one. And another.

I found myself wondering, *What is in that airplane? How does it fly anyway?*

When I trace the breadcrumbs that led to my becoming an aeronautical engineer, I think back to this moment, when fear transformed into love and terror morphed into curiosity.

Just look up.

I don't know that I realized then what a valuable skill that would be for me to carry through life. I was a person riddled with fear and anxiety. I've had many panic attacks in my life, and this one fear was just the beginning.

When I was in college doing research in the hypersonic shock tunnel, I had to climb down a swinging ladder into a twenty-feet-deep tank to change out a piece of my Scramjet model. I was paralyzed, stuck up on top of the tank, staring at the cheap, aluminum, swinging ladder for forty-five minutes, telling myself I had to do this. I told myself there was no way out, and I examined my fear just like in that mall parking lot. I looked at it.

Was it just the height? The fear of falling? The thought of the ladder breaking? The worry of slipping?

I decided it was a fear of my body weight breaking that cheesy, aluminum, swinging ladder. Fear of my work boots slipping off of the aluminum rungs. Fear of injury, falling, death. I talked to myself over and over.

The ladder is rated for my weight. I won't die. If I fall, it's not that far down.

Those fears were obvious, but what I didn't realize, what was way more subtle, was the fear of ridicule, embarrassment, scrutiny, and not living up to the mold of expectation that others felt for me. It only manifested in subtle ways I wasn't even aware of—until I looked.

Just look up. Or, in this case, down.

I placed a foot on the rung, then lifted it back up. Then again. Then two rungs down and back up, testing the ladder, the feel, my boots. Adrenaline pumping through my veins. My coworkers and other students kept walking by and asking if I was okay. I all but begged them to do this for me.

"Nope, you have to do it yourself."

I tried again, two or three rungs this time. Back up until I talked myself into it.

Face the fear. You can do this. It's going to be okay. You just did two or three rungs. One final push to get to the bottom.

The next thing I knew, I had made it to the bottom. I stood inside that red tank, huffing and puffing. I got my backpack off and changed my model. And then I climbed back up. Afterward, I felt so accomplished and proud of myself. During all my research, I completed this task hundreds more times, and each time, it got easier and easier.

This tool followed me throughout life. As an adult still struggling decades later with her weight, I found a fear buried in there, too—a fear that wasn't mine—a fear of being skinny. I didn't find that out until I got curious, until I looked.

Just look up.

An older couple across the street had egg-laying chickens, and one day in my teens, I went over there to help feed them. The rooster jumped on one of the scrawny hens. Her feathers were missing from being jumped on so much. I rolled my eyes and thought, *See, even the rooster likes skinny girls better! Everyone loves skinny girls.*

And then it dawned on me.

Maybe she's just easier to catch.

My brain latched onto that idea like the rooster to that chicken.

Are people more attracted to skinny girls just because they're more likely to be dominated and easier to catch, easier to rape? Is it a reptilian brain leftover? See, being fat is best, less likely to get jumped on.

And that, my friends, is how the conversation in my head works. The logic can mess you up. It may be highly logical, however we're now way more complex than a chicken, evolutionally. So I guess there's some probability that this theory isn't true, but it rang true to me.

Deep down in the darkness of my soul, getting skinny meant I was more likely to get raped. I believed skinny people get raped. A generational trauma passed down that was not mine, perhaps. A cultural innuendo spoken amongst older women around me. I am keenly aware that it significantly contributed to my not wanting to lose weight.

There has been so much pain and anxiety in my life about trying to get skinny, or to a healthy weight, or my natural weight. When I looked to see who I would be without this weight and who I would be if I were skinny, I couldn't visualize it. I realized I had a long way to go. Not just physically but emotionally and spiritually (energetically).

Who would I be without physical ailments like arthritis? Was I afraid of her? Was I afraid of her power? I was a little, but I'm not scared to look and see.

But I, as an adolescent girl facing her first big fear in the parking lot that day, had a long, long way to go.

CHAPTER 12

Under the Pink

I've got enough guilt to start my own religion.

–TORI AMOS

I started questioning the teachers in religious classes between fifth and eighth grade. For me, it was a significant age of awakening, an awakening of my intuition like Tori Amos' album *Under the Pink*, though I had no idea what to call it then. We would read a story from the Bible, and I would be like –

WHAT? Why is no one else questioning this craziness? Something doesn't seem right here. How can we all be from Adam and Eve? That doesn't make any sense. I thought you couldn't genetically marry your siblings, or you'd have freaky things happen, yet we're all descendants of some sibling craziness?

I wasn't going to swallow the pill that women are the reason for all original sin. Why would anyone sacrifice a child or a goat or anything for a weird deity in the sky who tells you what's right and wrong? To my grammar school brain, it sounded like maybe the guy had schizophrenia.

One day, the teacher left the room, and I started talking to the other seventh graders about how this was all a sham.

Someone said, "You're going to burn in hell if you put the Bible on the floor and step on it."

And so I did.

See? I'm not burning!

Maybe I will someday. Maybe my entire life's pain is my burning in hell. Maybe this is hell and heaven all mixed up because they're all words we assign subjectively.

Part of the problem was that my Catholic school hired teachers who didn't necessarily believe either. I can't be sure, but I felt my questions made some of them smile, like when your kids start questioning you about Santa Claus.

I never believed in Santa, either. I used to explain to my mom that we didn't even have a chimney, and the stuff looked like the stuff you could buy in a store, wrapped in the same wrapping paper she had in her closet.

So, I befriended those teachers, specifically my fifth-grade homeroom teacher, who also taught science to fifth through eighth graders. She also taught sex education and made sure we girls were all supported and felt like we had someone to talk to when we got our periods. She would referee when we were steeped in girl drama.

It wasn't just that I felt supported by her or had someone to talk to. It felt like she saw and appreciated who I was as a person. She was matter-of-fact and spoke in scientific language. She was fun. She let us sit with our friends in class instead of assigned seating. She was funny.

When one boy infuriated her, she slapped her hands together and said, "Watch me Irish temper."

We used to quote her all the time. I remember biking to her house in the summer and helping her plant flowers. Deep down, I related to the like-minded, scientific, matter-of-factness about her. She was the one who first taught me the scientific method. We had to make up an experiment, create a hypothesis, and conduct that experiment, and I remember feeling alive in the process.

I also loved my math teacher, who had the seventh-grade homeroom. She was taking a computer class outside of school and would come in and teach us what she learned. In early IBM days, the programs lived on 5.25-inch floppy disks, and you typed into the DIR in the DOS on monochrome monitors. We learned to program a little, and it was fun. I could express to Mrs. Remsen my desire to study something related to math and science in college, and she would listen.

This was the same time when the movie *Top Gun* came out. I didn't think about Tom Cruise or Val Kilmer. I wanted to fly those airplanes. I went to K-Mart and bought model airplanes. I found a poster of an F-14 Tomcat at Art Works in the Eastern Hills Mall, and it promptly went up on my pink rose wallpapered bedroom next to Michael Hutchence from INXS, River Phoenix, Kurt Cobain, and Keanu Reeves. Science, math, music, and F-14s became my world. I was starting to find my way.

Religion still didn't sit well with my insides. I hated religion class. It was like someone was speaking a different language. Oddly, I became involved in the church teen life group. This group sang more fun music and was led by an exceptional guy who was our new priest at the church, Father Larry. Even though I loved how young and hip Father Larry was and how he let us play electric guitar and real drums in the church band, I still knew.

I still knew deep down that Christianity wasn't for me.

Later, when I began questioning my religious beliefs even more, I wondered why I was so involved with the church at this time. I was confirmed and even became a Eucharistic minister. And yet, I didn't really believe it or admit that I didn't believe it.

I concluded that it was the people. So many churches have great communities. I wondered if Father Larry was still there, and if I stayed in East Amherst, would I have continued to go to church? Perhaps. Maybe I would have made peace with the evils of the Catholic religion and the patriarchy. But I doubt it.

I looked for the same type of community years later in life and even attended Bible study in towns that I moved to. I would question things, and everyone would just stare at me with no answers. I never found my fit in Christianity. I guess if you find your people, stay there. But for me, I'd take knowledge over ignorance any day.

CHAPTER 13

Fresh Blood

Your new life is going to cost you your old one.

–BRIANNA WIEST

In eighth grade, a girl in my class started cutting.

She cut cool designs into her thighs and showed us in the bathroom while we were changing for gym class. It wasn't a typical slashes-on-the-wrist, self-harm type of cutting. It was a cool-design, sort-of-like-a-tattoo cutting. So that made it seem okay. She carved names and symbols from bands into her skin, which I thought was cool. She said you could add color, and it would be like a free tattoo.

At this point, I had my own room. My aunt had moved out of the house, and my mom had taken her room, which meant we were across the hall from each other. She still worked a lot, so I was alone.

One afternoon, I went to the basement and got a straight razor from my grandpa's toolbox. I brought it upstairs into my bedroom, undressed, and started cutting into my thighs. I cut a peace sign, INXS, and a heart. It stung. The blood ran, but nothing excessive like a period—just one or two tissues-worth.

I bandaged them up and went to school. I changed in the stall the first few days so no one would see. By the time they healed, I showed them off, cool-looking scabs that would soon be scars. I still don't know who, but someone told on me.

Sister Sheila brought me to the convent, a house between the school and the church near the rectory where the priest lived. She made me pull up my skirt and show her my cuts. She was horrified and pressed for answers, but I didn't rat anyone out. She called my mom, and we had to talk that night. Nothing came of it.

In hindsight, I did get off on the cutting and did it a few more times. I can't explain the feeling or reason for doing it. I think it was a little bit of adrenaline. The pain made me focus on something different from the day-to-day. I didn't do it to punish myself. I never did it excessively, but I do understand its draw. And I feel for those who struggle with the habit. I can see how, like other habits, it's an outward way to soothe yourself when you don't know how to soothe internally.

I think about what I needed at that moment. Perhaps therapy would have helped, but it was never suggested. So I cut.

CHAPTER 14

Wild Boys

She will run wild with you, beside you… but let me tell you…
Love her wild or leave her there.

–NIKKI ROWE

My interest in boys started early. I was in love with the boy who lived behind my house at age four. He was (and still is) very attractive. He was one of my neighborhood best friends. We ran in the backyard, flew down the slip-n-slide, tore through the woods, zoomed on our bikes, and sliced through the snow on our sleds in the winter.

When I found out that he was having a birthday party and I didn't get invited, I punched him in the nose. After I did it, he told me his mom had said he couldn't invite girls. I immediately felt sorry.

We were supposed to kiss in the woods behind our house. We planned to meet, showed up, and chickened out. Later that day, in my driveway, I gave him a peck on the cheek, and it was over. I think I was five.

My mom used to say, "School is for school. Stop looking at the boys!"

I can see now, after a lot of wrong turns, how right she was. I didn't know then that the obsession with boys would be like choosing to go into the black hole, like Sarah when she fell into the helping hands hole in *Labyrinth*.

One day, a boy in my kindergarten class asked me and another girl if he could look up our skirts

With little hesitation, we said, "Sure. Why not?"

I thought he was weird for wanting to do it, and I knew it was bad and wrong. But I let him do it anyway. I didn't feel shame; I felt excitement. It was yet another sin I never confessed.

The sins were soon to stack up.

One boy, let's call him Jay, was a year younger than me and was a cutie pie. We sat on the bus together and talked about *Encyclopedia Brown* books, F-14s, and skateboards. I couldn't believe he wanted to talk to me. I couldn't believe he was sitting with me.

It was fifth grade, and we started dating. Back then, dating consisted of writing notes, and ours were always about *Top Gun*. I called him on the phone. I knew where he lived, so I rode my bike to his house. He promised he would take me to the restaurant Ponderosa on our first real date. He said he would let me ride with him on his skateboard. I was head over heels in love, and I felt so special.

Two weeks later, he started dating Ann.

It felt like the floor dropped out from under me and another cinder block jammed into the wall that was steadily building around my heart. The message was clear. Don't trust boys. Don't trust your best friend.

Why does this keep happening? Why do I not see it coming? My mind raced, trying to make sense of the betrayal.

I never spoke to him again. I didn't even blame him or Ann. I thought immediately, *Well, that tracks. I'm not good enough.*

I moved on, and later I started to become obsessed with a new boy who came to our little Catholic school in seventh grade. Let's call him Charles. Charles had a weird scar on his face that intrigued me. He was quiet. His little brother started at the same time, and the school was abuzz. We heard they were adopted.

I never told him how much I liked him, so nothing happened. We didn't have a friendship, but I stared at him and swore he would stare back at me. I always spoke about him to Ann, and in hindsight, she rarely commented.

She didn't agree with me when I talked about him, but she also didn't *disagree* or assert that he wasn't hot.

"Did you see him look at me today when I flinched," I'd say. "Did you see what he did at lunch?"

She kept quiet.

Ann and I were getting ready for the eighth-grade dance, an event at the school hall right after church and our graduation ceremony. There was dinner and then a dance. Family members were asked to attend, and I invited my mom, Grandpa, Aunt Frannie and Ellie, and Grandma K.

Charles's handsome older brother danced with me a couple of times. In hindsight, I wonder if he was trying to keep me away from Charles. At the end of the dance, we packed up and were ready to leave. I left the hall and saw Charles kissing Ann in the parking lot. My stomach dropped out, and the world began to spin again.

More proof. Trust no one. Another cinder block. Another wall.

Jay and Charles were just the first. I thought about boys all the time. I wanted to kiss their faces, hold hands, and do everything I saw on TV. I thought about them in church and in my bed. I was masturbating before I knew what I was doing and what it was, and thankfully, I never felt guilty about that.

Little did I know I'd go from a potential bad girl in a Catholic school to an actual bad girl in real life.

CHAPTER 15

Having Tea with the Devil

Shadow work is the path of the heart warrior.

−CG JUNG

I watched a lot of television when I was young. You could say the TV was a bit of a babysitter.

The original Nickelodeon and *You Can't Do That on Television*. *Sesame Street, Electric Company*, Saturday morning cartoons, Sunday evening *Hee Haw* and *The Muppet Show*, sitcoms, news, *Jeopardy*. A lot of NBC movies like *North and South* with Patrick Swayze. After we got cable, I would tape all sorts of movies.

One NBC miniseries in 1987 called *Billionaire Boys Club* documented the actual Billionaire Boys Club from the 1970s in Southern California. One scene in that show fundamentally changed how I looked at the world and made sense of why we believe what we believe. (Ironically, my big life lesson from TV had to be from a show about a boys club, of all things.)

In the program, Judd Nelson's character defines a paradigm shift for his friend. He explains that a piece of paper could be black on one side and white on the other. You can see the white, and I can see the black. As we look at it, we're both arguing about the color of the piece of paper, and we're both right. Then someone turns the paper, and you can see it's white on one side and black on the other. The veil is taken down. You realize that you were both wrong and both right. You see what the other person sees as if walking in their shoes. You wake up to what's real, and your eyes are opened. This is a paradigm shift.

As individuals, we view the world using the model our brains built based on our experiences—an algorithm. It's a way we can sort, categorize, and compartmentalize what we see, feel, and experience. We each define right and wrong subconsciously, and when someone opens the door to seeing things in a new and different way, the model is changed. The algorithm leverages more data. Learning begets more paradigm shifts if we're open to it.

When we tell someone they are wrong, we argue that the sheet of paper is not two-sided. If we could get curious about what the other person sees, maybe we wouldn't have such staunch dualities in our society, like right versus left. Perhaps instead of arguing our point, we could first ask why or how the other person is arguing their point. What would it be like if we did that? This concept unlocked an entire wing of the labyrinth for me. It was a key in my pocket that would continue to open locks to new doors as I traversed the maze throughout life.

Once this veil dropped, my teenage brain was consumed with the human psyche. I became obsessed with the Metallica song "One" and explored death and existence. I read the book *Johnny Got His Gun* and watched the movie repeatedly. It's about a man who is severely wounded in war. His legs, arms, eyes, ears, and vocal cords are all damaged, but his mind is alive. He can feel the nurses coming into the hospital. The book and the movie go through him waking up and realizing what has happened to him. In the end, he uses his head to spell out "kill me" in Morse code.

I was also taken with the movie *Flatliners*. I wished I could do what they did and die momentarily to see what it was like. This spawned more research into psychological manipulation. While this may seem strange and unusual for an eighth-grade girl to be interested in, it brought me great satisfaction to understand how the mind works, what manipulation is, and what drives people. In a way, it was a path for healing, to understand people have very good reasons for doing what they do, and it might (usually) not have anything to do with me.

I think it's important to allow yourself to dive into the depths of what you want to explore. Like facing fear, you have to face darkness, looking at the shadow sides of your personality and shining light on them. My teenage years were filled with exploring those dark arts, and they were terrific lessons I never would have learned if I hadn't let myself go there. I was interested in goth music, ordered black-out catalogs, bought fishnet stockings, wore Doc Martens, and listened to Sisters of Mercy. My mom was horrified when I hung a black rosary around my neck. She would talk to me about the music I was listening to. My grandpa felt bad for me because he thought I had to wear Doc Martens as corrective shoes.

I laughed and told him, "No, Grandpa, these are cool."

While this dark exploration soothed my soul, I still didn't know who or what my identity was. I still struggled when I had to fill out college or work forms. Do I choose the "white Caucasian" box? Do I pick "other?" I didn't feel it was ever appropriate to select "Hispanic." I wasn't raised Hispanic, and I didn't speak Spanish. I was raised German and even minored in it in college.

So, where did I fit?

CHAPTER 16

Politically Correct High School

There are no rules if you're a boy. If you're a girl,
you have to play the game.

–MADONNA

I love the energy of newness, exploring, and learning. Big cities, universities, and places where there are lots of people, especially new people, all thrill me. That was the feeling I got when I walked into Williamsville North High School. It was modern, clean, and BIG. I went from Catholic school with the same class of about fifteen to public high school with a class of about 240. It was awesome. Lockers and sports teams. A real band. Bio lab, chem lab, computers. A real gym and a pool.

Though my high school was public, a relatively wealthy area in a suburb of Buffalo called Williamsville. Williamsville schools were considered top-notch, and much of the area housed professors from the University at Buffalo as well as players for the Sabres and the Bills. Our high school was said to have seventy-two different religious denominations. I was floored that there were even that many different religions. I felt like I had led such a previously sheltered life. I mean, I had no idea. Other than my uncle complaining about being laid off because the Jewish people took over his store and having one friend in dance who was Protestant (I remember asking my mom what that meant), I didn't have any idea that there were so many other diverse religions. I was pissed and felt betrayed by my family and Catholic school that they hadn't taught me about the real world.

I took flute lessons during grammar school, but I wasn't very good. In high school, I was in the seventeenth seat, the last person. Our band director, Mr. Ray, asked if any flute players would be willing to switch to trombone. Two of us, the last two seats, raised our hands. I loved the trombone and Mr. Ray. He was a charismatic person, and I enjoyed the lessons with him. He was so passionate about band that it was infectious. We all had the assignment to go to a concert or show once a quarter and write up who we saw, what they performed, how it was, etc. He told me about the Eastman School of Music and how they had a trombone choir. I went to see them and continued to return to Eastman for more concerts in the future.

One day, when I arrived for my lesson, Mr. Ray complained about having to change some songs for the holiday show to be more accommodating and politically correct.

"Pretty soon, all we are going to have is vanilla Jell-O," he grumbled.

That was the first time I had heard the expression "politically correct." I listened to him complain but realized how it must make people feel to be excluded. I didn't like his term vanilla Jell-O. It pissed me off. And so, I wrote a poem about it. It was later published—my first published poem.

After my encounter with Mr. Ray, I never assumed anyone's religion. If there were any reason to know, I would ask people what their religion was instead of assuming. I remember sitting next to a Muslim friend in class who was celebrating Ramadan, and I was fascinated. I wanted to know the history, the reasons for the fasting, how her family celebrated, how it differed, or if everyone did it the same. The vastness of variety was amazing. There was another student who was Buddhist and another Zen. I wasn't close enough to them to be asking them their business, so I looked it up in the library. Even though my excitement and curiosity were at an all-time high, I obliged my mother and grandfather, continued attending church, and continued going to CCD.

I was still in Girl Scouts through high school, and we once attended a cultural event in downtown Buffalo. The Indian man in all white doing yoga enthralled me. I ate tabbouleh and hummus for the first time. I felt like my whole body was resonating. I felt at home.

In high school, I knew I loved science and math, and I wanted to consume it all. I took a quiz in the career center that said I should be an aircraft mechanic. This didn't seem right to me. I turned up my nose because I wanted to be a pilot or design aircraft.

Because I came from a private school, I was behind. Some kids had the opportunity to take ninth-grade math, science, English, and social studies in eighth grade. The intelligent, more advanced kids were ahead. So I mapped out what classes I could take in the summers to catch up to them—health and social studies, and I could double up on math and science during the school year to take all of the AP classes Williamsville North offered. And so I did. I built my own curriculum with little to no advice from anyone. I asked the questions. I did the work. I was driven. My love of science, math, and fighter jets pointed me on the right path for my life.

While the religion thing still wasn't sitting well with me, science and math were the logic and music to my ears that made the world make sense. They were calming and reassuring. The scientific method of creating a hypothesis, testing it, statistically analyzing the data, and realizing the caveat that it only applies to this one environment in which you took the data made me realize the errors of our human ways. It was a perfect explanation for why people have so many opinions. Their data is real, but most don't realize the caveat that it only applies to them.

Opinions are like assholes; everyone has one.

I'm unsure where I first heard that one, but it's a funny recap of this theory. Your experiences are real data points, but recognizing that they are a data point of one is essential for compassion. We may find others with the same or a similar data points, and so we believe from two or three that it applies to the world. And then we offer advice based on that. If we all came to realize and awaken to the reality that we do this (offer our own advice) and also be able to recognize when people are giving us advice as their truth, they are doing it out of a data point of one.

Just because your data proves something works for you, and now it's a belief for you, doesn't mean it will work for everyone or anyone else. Realizing this was one big key to solving the labyrinth and eventually taking the walls down, though using that key took me a while. While these religions and experiences broadened my horizons, they made me realize that Christianity may not be the right path for me, and maybe that was okay.

Vanilla Jell-O

Die, or be
exactly as you are
told to be
There is no original,
unique, independence
Nothing is yours
It's just an illusion
you view through
your vanilla Jell-O
Trademark America
the man
the burning man even
has rules, regulations
safety.
You do not exist until
you are one of the
crowd, and then you
do not exist because
you are the crowd.
Die, or be.
There is no other option.

CHAPTER 17

Concertgoers

Ah, music…A magic beyond all we do here!

–JK ROWLING, *HARRY POTTER AND THE SORCERER'S STONE*

In the midst of it all, there was music. In the bad times, it consoled me. When the demons came into my head, music was my paradigm shift. It was and continues to be a huge part of my life.

It all started with my best friend Ann and her siblings. Her older sister was into new wave music. Living in Buffalo, we could get the alternative station broadcasted from the top of the CN tower in Toronto, and I used my boombox to record songs from the radio show.

In fourth grade, Ann called me on the phone and said, "You have to come over here and see this guy's crazy hair on this music video!"

I went over and watched her sister's VCR tape of The Cure. Ann and her mom were laughing.

"Can you believe this guy's hair?" they cackled.

I was mesmerized by Robert Smith. "But I really like this music," I kept saying.

I remember Ann being obsessed with INXS—the *Shabooh Shoobah* album. I decided to try out my aunt's records. She had The Fixx, Journey, Phil

Collins, and Michael Jackson.

The first tape I bought was Michael Jackson because I didn't know any better. This was back when there was a mail-in order deal where you got ten records or tapes for free, with an obligation to buy ten more over ten months. It was the best. I grew my record collection quickly. I thought I would like some based on the covers, like Poison, but I ended up hating them.

My uncle took me to my first concert, the Beach Boys, and he made me copies of his Beatles albums. I quickly loved concerts, and my mom took Ann and me to many. I have fond memories of my mom dragging me to concerts all over Buffalo (King Swamp in some bar, Bare Naked Ladies in multiple bars in Elmwood, and visiting the old Darien Lake amphitheater). Decades later, I would keep the tradition alive and drag my own son and his friends to see Green Day.

Ann's taste started to drift from mine. She liked rap and pop, specifically New Kids on the Block (NKOTB). I didn't enjoy listening to them, but I thought Joey was cute. I liked LL Cool J, too. I bought their albums, but mostly I loved putting on records of Depeche Mode, New Order, Sinead O'Connor, and Sisters of Mercy. There was one girl in high school who was very goth, and I befriended her. She introduced me to Suzie and the Banshees.

While Ann and I started to explore and make friends in high school, we met a group of nice girls who also loved NKOTB. They were obsessed. I thought it was funny, but I also felt bad when they were made fun of. I didn't like that music, but they were my friends, so I begrudgingly tagged along to many concerts with them and even started tolerating some of their favorite bands. I thought Marky Mark and the Funky Bunch was way better than NKOTB, and I enjoyed C&C Music Factory. Part of me was grumpy about always seeing bands I didn't love, but in hindsight, I'm glad I didn't just dismiss these girls based on our differences. Their friendship meant a lot to me and still does. We see each other now (mostly at funerals and reunions), and it's always good to catch up.

John was another friend I grew closer to because of music. We had grown up in the same church, but it wasn't until I transferred to his public high school that we became friends. He always hated Ann and me because he thought we were snobby rich kids who went to Catholic school. Funny enough, we were the poor ones. We thought John was stuck up because he lived in the rich developments around our house. After we broke through all the judgment and ignoring each other in the hallways, we found out we were both pretty okay. John played the bassoon in band, and although I didn't sit next to him, he was one of the few friends I had in band. We got closer when we played switch band and got to teach each other our instruments. He lived only about half a mile away, and we started hanging out—rollerblading, playing cards, talking about music.

John had no music knowledge at first. Then he started working at Record Town and eventually knew more than me. We shared our dieting adventures and mishaps and would skip school to go to Burger King and get chicken sandwiches. John later confided in me that he was gay, and I was so happy that I was one of the first people he told. John and I went to Green Day, Tori Amos, and Depeche Mode. To this day, we are still friends and still go to concerts together. I am forever grateful for his friendship.

Everything Counts

I'm taking a ride with my best friend
I don't want to put my feet back down on the ground
If you tried walking in my shoes
You might stumble in my footsteps
But I know the policy of truth

I hear you speak to me

And I enjoy the silence

You see, people are people
Who just can't get enough
Grabbing hands grab all they can
Is it just a question of lust?

In your room I'm stripped down to my bones
And I'll wag my tongue
When everything is dark

It is all of these things and more that keep us together

Enough is enough

Everything counts in large amounts

This precious life
I've been waiting for the night for so long
My cosmos, my personal Jesus
I look to you, how you carry on, because another angel has died
The world in my eyes
And when I squinted the world is rose-tinted

CHAPTER 18

Hold My Ice Cream

You don't have to be pretty. You don't owe prettiness to anyone.
Not to your boyfriend/spouse/partner, not to your coworkers, especially not
to random men on the street. You don't owe it to your mother, you don't owe
it to your children, you don't owe it to civilization in general.
Prettiness is not a rent you pay for occupying a space marked 'female.'

–ERIN MCKEAN

I fueled myself in high school with pure shit. Cookies, buttered rolls, pizza, and ice cream. Surprisingly, I didn't gain much weight. I entered high school at a size eighteen and stayed there nearly the entire time. I rarely brought my lunch, instead choosing from the indulgent cafeteria options.

Monitoring my food intake and dieting were not my focus in high school. I was having so much fun learning and exploring new things that the pain of being fat and focusing on what I was eating was only a small, constant undertone compared to other times in my life. My size was beneficial when we played basketball in gym class and in the weight room. I didn't do many sports in high school. I thought about continuing softball but was too afraid. Ann and I joined the tennis team, but we were last string and typically played together. I joined the rifle team, but it wasn't very athletic.

Even though I wasn't as interested in boys as I was when I was younger, I did think one of the basketball players was super cute. He would smile at me in the hall, and I'd smile back. One day, I was sitting in the cafeteria with friends, eating an ice cream bar. Our books and homework were all over the table, and we were chatting. I saw this boy come into the cafeteria. I didn't want him to see me eating ice cream, so I put it under the table. I was trying to get my friend to hold or take it from me. He called me over, and since I couldn't get her attention, I put it on her leg. She flipped out and screamed and totally blew my cover. I gave her wide eyes and quietly yelled under my breath what I was doing and why. She just shook her head and threw my ice cream away.

I was embarrassed with my food choices, yet I kept doing it. Geneen Roth proposes that people with food issues are either "permitters" or "restrictors." I was definitely a "permitter." When around comfortable people like friends and family, I would permit myself to eat anything. I'd permit you to as well. I was the life of the party, feeding everyone tons of good food. I still do this. Restrictors typically turn to anorexia and OCD, counting each calorie, compulsively re-measuring, and restricting until the point of a binge primarily based on bodily need.

My food issues were pervasive throughout my life and ultimately kept me from being a fighter pilot.

Resistance

Sabotage Monster
is too tired
Tried once before and didn't work
Can't
need chocolate
need something
ate last night
fuck it
stressed
who cares
 let's party

CHAPTER 19

Put a CAP in It

Each time a woman stands up for herself, without knowing it possibly,
without claiming it, she stands up for all women.

—MAYA ANGELOU

During high school, I joined the Civil Air Patrol (CAP), an auxiliary of the U.S. Air Force for high school students. We got to wear Air Force-issue blues and camos. My mom drove me to Rome, New York, at Griffiss Air Force Base, the closest Air Force base to our house, to pick up my uniforms. This was my ticket to gain an ROTC scholarship and then become a fighter pilot or astronaut, although more of the U.S. Navy flies fighters than the Air Force. The Air Force has more cargo and reconnaissance aircraft. I spent hours learning drill, learning how to debate, and listening to lectures from pilots who have served or were actively serving.

I attended two New York State Civil Air Patrol encampments, and they were life-changing. The first was an emergency services encampment that included learning how to communicate on the radio, orienteering, survival skills, and navigation. Part of the mission of the Civil Air Patrol was to help in cases of mass emergency services. For example, the Civil Air Patrol helped scour the fields of Texas, Louisiana, and Oklahoma to find pieces and parts of the NASA Columbia space shuttle that deteriorated on re-entry in 2003. So, going to the emergency service encampment was training for such an event.

The days were filled with jumping out of the bunk, making the bed, brushing my teeth, and getting dressed for physical training (PT) within two minutes. We'd head outside for PT, then shower, eat breakfast, and attend classes all day. The encampment was on an actual Air Force base. On the last day, we were rewarded with an open-door Huey (Bell H-1) helicopter flight.

I also went to a leadership encampment on the Plattsburgh Air Force base the same week in the summer that my Girl Scout troop was going to Disneyland. Yep, I chose to go to a week-long encampment that included getting up and doing PT before the real Air Force boot camp cadets over Disneyland. This encampment had a lot of outdoor drills in the very hot summer as well as indoor classroom activities.

We were taught how to make hospital corners on our beds, shine our shoes, and keep our rooms perfectly neat. We were told to carry a little blue book with the rules and three demerits. The demerits could be pulled at any time by any officer for something good or bad, but mostly bad. They could pull demerits for unshined shoes, not knowing the rules, having an unclean room, not following orders, etc. The demerits could also be pulled for good things like showing leadership or helping others. The fear drove compliance. I liked the structure.

I liked the 5 a.m. Reveille bugle call. When it went off, you had two minutes to pee, brush your teeth, get dressed, and be lined up for PT in the hall. You slept in your PT gear with shoes at the end of the bed and your toothbrush on the dresser next to you. PT was difficult for me, not having any physical fitness. We were supposed to run a mile each morning with the whole "flight" (the rest of my group), but I never could keep up. I always had to stop, walk, and hang my head in shame, watching the flight take off ahead of me in unison. The push-ups and sit-ups were okay, but running was my weakness.

One humid morning, a leader from another flight stayed with me. I don't remember his name, but I felt like he was the nicest person in the world. When everyone else ignored me, he helped me. He ran with me and guided me to slow down my breathing.

"Breathe in for three steps—right, left, right. Breathe out for three steps —left, right, left. Don't sprint," he instructed. "Just jog. Control. Then endure."

I finished the whole mile that day. At lunch, the leader of the entire encampment approached me. When an officer approaches you, you stand up. I was nervous, thinking she would quiz me on the blue book rules. She asked for one of my demerits and took it for my efforts that morning in PT.

"Thank you, ma'am," I said with shy happiness.

I sat back down and continued eating my hardened Jell-O squares and tuna casserole lunch. It was a pivotal moment in my athletic career.

Am I a runner? Did I do a good thing?

Every moment before this, I hated everything to do with running and being an athlete. I hated missing the swings at Catholic school. I hated running for softball. I hated track. I never felt like an athlete and definitely never felt like a runner. It was a thorn in my side up until that point. I still wasn't an athlete, but at that moment, I felt like it was possible. I wanted to master running. I wanted to like it. I wanted to overcome the frustration. I had made a tiny bit of progress, and I wanted more.

Contradictions

I own a gun.

I was on the rifle team.

My husband hunts.

I like target practice.

And.

I believe we need more gun control.

Accept the contradiction. It's okay. Let it go. They can co-exist.

I work for an aerospace company.

I support the war fighter.

I love these aircraft.

And.

I believe humanity has a real possibility to create a future where our emotional bodies are guides for a positive future to overcome issues without war, without fear-based decisions. This may take hundreds of years, but one certainly can visualize this future state.

Accept the contradiction. It's okay. Let it go. They can co-exist.

Stay informed.

Vote.

Know the issues.

Understand the risks.

Educate yourself.

Speak up.

Join a revolution.

And.

Take care of your sanity, turn off the news, balance screen time, come back to community, question what is shoved down your throat. Prep and feed the chickens. Dry some oranges. Make Christmas gifts instead of buying them from China.

Accept the contradiction. It's okay. Let it go. They can co-exist.

Eat this. I made it for you.

Love is pumpkin bread and apple pie and we go out for ice cream and birthday cakes.

The booze flows at parties and weekends and then nightly.

Wine and meal pairings.

Eat the pop tarts and pita bread and hummus, alcohol and donut holes.

And.

Sugar and alcohol are the number one cause of cancer and aging. They are drugs to numb. Eliminate. Fast. Keto.

Accept the contradiction. It's okay. Let it go. They can co-exist.

Do the laundry.

Work ten hours a day.

Cook beautiful healthy meals.

Have perfect, well-behaved, well-rounded, healthy children.

Do the mobility, strength, stretches, ultra marathon, triathlon, hike.

Be a good friend.

Have a good spiritual connection.

Perfect modern house with all the clear plastic containers showing all your stuff.

And.

I can't, it's too much, you have to do it all. Fear. Worry. Comparison.

Accept the contradiction. It's okay. Let it go. They can co-exist.

I want to be acknowledged.

I want to be wanted.

I want attention.

I want to be loved.

I want to be right.

And.

There's too much chaos for anyone to care. I married a man who doesn't show verbal affection. I'm tired of people telling me what to do. Mom always being right. I want to be alone and solo car camp with my dog.

Accept the contradiction. It's okay. Let it go. They can co-exist.

There seems to be a revolution where we are evolving, getting real awareness of what our feelings are and learning to heal generational trauma, and learning how to communicate, give corrective action, learn unconscious bias in a way that's not hurtful towards others.

And.

The trolls are getting louder. The ignorance is getting worse. I worry about a civil war.

Accept the contradiction. It's okay. Let it go. They can co-exist.

CHAPTER 20

Grandma

Forgiveness is a gift you give yourself.

–SUZANNE SOMERS

When I was sixteen, I started working at a local grocery store called Tops at the corner of Maple and Transit in Amherst. I was the bottle girl counting dirty, gross cans and bottles for NY $0.05 return. I surprisingly really liked this job. It was simple, somewhat physical, and satisfying. I got kudos for how clean I kept the area. There were giant bins for the two-liters, containers for the cans, boxes for the glass, a cart for the beer cases, and another cart for the longneck soda eight- and twelve-packs. When the cart got full, you had to roll them to the back of the store and throw the big bags of two-liters in a two-story bin. When I first started, I couldn't get the bags up over the wall, and soon I was throwing them without looking, sometimes two at a time. I mopped the floor and cleaned the counters. To this day, I love the smell of rotten beer and sticky soda cans when I return mine.

The bottle desk was attached to the customer service desk, and if I had no work, I could talk to the service desk folks. I aspired and eventually was asked to move up to the service desk, which was also a mindless yet satisfying job that I used to describe as playing Monopoly. I convinced Ann and other friends to work at Tops. I made lifetime friends. I gained the independence I so desperately sought.

One day, my mom and a police officer (a co-worker and friend of my mom's and someone I used to babysit for) came into the store.

"Honey, you have to come with me. Something happened to Grandma."

"What happened?!" My mind raced.

"Just come with me," she said firmly.

I nervously walked over to the service desk and told them I had to leave for a family emergency. I went in the back, clocked out, took my apron off, walked around to the front, and met my mom. It was a bright, sunny day, and leaving Tops and going outside hurt my eyes. I slid into the back seat of the cop car with my mom.

"Grandma passed away. We're going to the hospital."

I couldn't process this news. I kept slapping my face and pinching myself to wake up.

"No, no, no," I repeated it over and over again.

The news was too big for me to process. I didn't cry. I was in shock.

We walked into Millard Fillmore Hospital into a tiny room where my grandfather was. Grandpa was hard of hearing, and when the doctor told him that she had passed, he didn't hear what he'd said. I had to repeat it for him.

"Oh," he said. He held me tight, and I think he cried. I was more sad for him than me.

My mom said Grandma had passed out, and Grandpa had called 911 while my mom was working. They took Grandma in the ambulance to the hospital and tried to resuscitate her on the way, but she didn't make it. We were ushered into a dark room where the lights were turned off. With only ambient light trickling in, we said our goodbyes to her cold, dead body.

I just looked at her. No feelings.

I still had the hate in my heart. I wasn't sad. I wasn't relieved. I wasn't happy. I felt bad for Grandpa. He truly loved her, and he was heartbroken. I was sad for my mom, who was crying. I knew this would be a fundamental shift in our home life, and I was scared about that.

Later, after I made peace with Grandma during many years of therapy, my mom told me nice stories about her. She told me she was pretty normal when she was little. She remembered Grandma having her first nervous breakdown when my mom was eleven or twelve. She remembered how much she loved to cook and bake and how she got so many compliments for how good her food was.

She told me stories about Grandma working at George Urban's. She would cook all the food for the hunters who came in and was always complimented on her work. I later looked up the history of George Urban, and I could picture my grandma, hair done up in a bouffant, perfect apron, sprinkling paprika and placing parsley leaves on a German potato salad.

She was with me and is with me many days, especially days I feel like cooking or baking. Her true self. Her authentic self. May she rest in peace.

CHAPTER 21

Tituba

They were not witches; they were women.

—MINNIE IN *TRIFLES*

Our high school had a great drama club and a number of talented perform-
ing arts teachers, and our school plays and musicals were very well done. I
always auditioned and sometimes made it in the chorus or the pit, but never
a lead…

Until I played Tituba in *The Crucible* as a senior.

Tituba was an enslaved person who was thought to have been from Bar-
bados, owned by the Parris family in colonial Massachusetts, and the first to
be accused in the Salem Witch Trials. Even though *The Crucible* is a fiction-
alized story of the trials, Tituba was real.

At the time, I was somewhat upset that I was cast in this part because
she was a dark-skinned, big woman with a funny accent. Of course, I was
cast as the big woman. Tituba worked as a slave, cooking, cleaning, and taking care of the Parris children. I was grumpy, but I decided to own the part,
to fully embrace this and the experience.

Since Tituba was thought to have taught all of the women of Salem
witchcraft, the director of the play wanted to start the show with the curtains

closed and me on the stage above a staircase that went down into the open space of the auditorium where a cauldron would be set up. The lights would go down, and I'd walk on stage and take my spot. The native tribal music would start, and the spotlight would go on me. I would dance a bit on stage and then dance down the stairs and make a gesture to call all of the women from the forest. The other girls in the play would be scattered throughout the dark auditorium amongst the guests. They would rise up and meet me at the cauldron. We would dance around the cauldron, and I would give one of the girls a chalice. She would pretend to drink, bite into a fake blood capsule, and then face the audience with blood dripping down her chin.

The director told me to act like I owned it. Dance my heart out. Be in my body. I didn't know how to do this. I practiced and practiced, but it was still so mechanical. I wasn't losing it to the music. I wasn't letting it flow. I wasn't in my power. He kept working with me, and eventually I got a glimpse of what he meant.

Little did I know this was a prelude, a big sign pointing me in a direction, a sign from the Universe. I didn't know I am my version of Tituba in real life. Playing the role allowed me to take up space, be in my body, and get in touch with the earth and the world. I didn't know I had the power to lead, affect change, and gather women. It was a tiny prelude that would take years to develop and for me to learn my power. I would learn to defeat the patriarchy many times over and maybe get beaten by them, but not killed, not yet.

I bonded with the rest of the cast and spent all my free time in the band room, the auditorium, at rehearsals, and watching the scene designers bring the show to life. I fell in love with another cast member during this play. He played one of the other characters, a judge. We would sneak away to the top of the auditorium and watch the rehearsal, holding hands, touching knees, him playing with my hair. We were never really officially boyfriend/girlfriend, but we hung out all the time, even after the play was over.

I helped him with his make-up the night of the play, and he did mine. I asked him to go with me to he prom, and he said yes. I was over the moon, even though his parents were not all that excited. We had the best time at the prom, dancing and kissing on the dance floor. I spent the summer still pining over him and hung out at his house a few times. When I went away to college and came back to him at the first break, we still had fun together, but after the next break and by the next summer, he had another new girlfriend. Years later, I found out on Facebook that he was gay. I will forever be happy for his love and affection.

The play was an important moment in my life. I tasted a small sampling of my power and what it could feel like to embrace my body. I found companionship with a boy and felt safe in my skin with him. But most importantly, I realized through Tituba that it wasn't witches who were burned; it was women. It was women who were beaten into submission, expressing their attempt to save each other. And as a woman, I felt a fire light in me through playing that role. Like Sarah slowly shifting from victim to victor throughout *Labyrinth*, playing Tituba was a powerful pivot point for me. And even though it would take me many more years to understand and activate that power, it was an important beginning.

PART 3

Wandering My Labyrinth

CHAPTER 22

Wild Oats

We were all sluts in the '90s.

–CHERYL STRAYED

When I told people I was going to Rensselaer Polytechnic Institute (RPI) to be an aeronautical engineer, they were like, "What?" They were shocked that I had chosen this path. Shocked that a female was doing that. I never quite knew whether to be happy or offended at the comments. So, of course, I kept quiet.

Besides participating in the Civil Air Patrol, I told no one about my aerospace obsession. I secretly used to go to the Amherst Library and check out Janes' books from the library. I secretly built model airplanes. I secretly watched old World War II History Channel shows. I kept it quiet. I'm not sure why. I thought no one would understand, except for that one boy in grade school and maybe my CAP people.

And later, that one man I dated from Ohio, a man who washed aircraft at the Fort Worth Air Force base. He understood my obsession with the fine lines. The beauty of the designs. Trying to understand why one fighter looked one way and the other looked another, arguing over which one was more aesthetically appealing. It's an obsession that Elon Musk, with his flush door handles, and Howard Hughes, with his flush rivets, would understand too. There's something magical about the soaring, sailplane-gliding, gravity-defying F-14 Tomcat. The wing movement. Not many people get me. So I kept it quiet.

I didn't want to stay home and go to University at Buffalo. I considered Clarkson, other State University of New York (SUNY) schools, and Maritime College in the Bronx. I regret never applying to MIT or any Ivy League schools. I felt like I would never get in, so I didn't bother. Since my high school was very elite, I ranked maybe forty-two out of around 200, and I felt inadequate compared to my peers.

I almost didn't go to RPI in Troy, New York. I declined because I thought I couldn't afford it. But then they called me up and offered me a free ride for the first two years and minimal tuition for the last two, assuming I kept a three-point grade point average or higher. I remember hemming and hawing about it and going to the high school guidance counselor. She said RPI was slightly more prestigious than Clarkson, which sealed the deal for me.

The RPI campus had a magical and historic feel. The architecture was a mixture of older, red brick buildings and a modern cement block library. They turned an old cathedral into the computing center, and a 1970s brown brick was the engineering center. The well-manicured landscape with cement circles to gather on made me happy. I loved the newness, the computer labs, the research, and the people. These were my people. Wind tunnels and machine shops. I was in second heaven.

I was assigned to live on the third floor in Nason Hall, which was all female. While the first two floors seemed to house the entire football team except for a small group of super smart, introverted engineers who brought printouts and digital copies of the previous programming code they had written home to impress everyone.

I struggled the first year at college primarily because of female relationships—more cinder blocks in the labyrinth walls. The girls and the gossip and fighting were ridiculous. The girl across the hall smoked pot daily (and ultimately flunked out), while another girl dated two men and tried to keep it from both of them. Another girl down the hall admitted that her only goal was to have sex with the entire hockey team.

The first two weeks were like the honeymoon period, and after that, it turned into drama central. It was like watching the *Bachelor* or *Love Is Blind*. I could write a whole book on the chaos of Nason 3—the nighttime sledding, the excessive drinking, and losing my virginity to a cute, deep-thinking hippie guy in my humanities class. The fire extinguisher and water wars, the backstabbing bitches, the girls who never spoke to anyone, my first sexual encounter with a girl on the eve before a break, throwing a pie in the face of a guy who told everyone I slept with him when all I did was give him a blow job on his sorry, small, limp dick.

Later, I would see him passing in the hall with his girlfriend, and she was so smug, her face saying, "Haha, I got him."

I thought, *Girl, I know what you got, and I think I won and dodged that bullet.*

My roommate was an Indian girl who was pre-med. She was doing three years at RPI and three years at the University of Albany, followed by residency. She was very religious and practiced her harpsichord before her Sikhism service on Sundays. I loved listening to her play (albeit I was always a little hungover). She made wonderful-smelling Indian food.

In the beginning, we got along, as I was curious about her, her religion, and her upbringing. She seemed kind, but we didn't have a lot in common. We went to a Diwali festival together, but our friendship ended shortly after that. She was conceited and tried to mother me, so we did not get along. I ran hard and fast away from being told what to do, and I wouldn't take it. I told her how I felt once, and she backed off. We remained courteous and distant to one another.

I'm a little sad we couldn't get past our friction and be friends. Once, when I was in grad school, I ran into her in the library and tried to make amends, but she would not let down her guard enough to be a real person. I think she had a lot of family pressure and expectations she put on herself and wasn't all that happy.

A slightly stocky girl from New Jersey—let's call her Amanada—asked me if I wanted to do crew with her. It was a resounding yes for me. I had heard that the president of the college wanted to make RPI into an Ivy League school and said we needed a crew team. The team was pretty sparse, maybe sixteen to twenty people. We practiced every weekday and on Saturdays. We would wake up at four-thirty in the morning, walk to the Union, and get a ride to the boathouse, which was on Troy's wastewater treatment facility on the Hudson River. The following year, the boathouse was moved to share with the State University of New York (SUNY) Albany right in downtown Albany.

In the beginning, I would follow the incumbent crew members, grabbing paddles and walking them down to the dock, picking up a crew boat with others, putting it on our shoulders, walking it down the floating docks, picking it up again, and rolling it over our heads and into the water. The boat was heavy, and we walked with the rim on our shoulders. Once in the water, there was a little one-foot-sized pedestal to get into the boat and sit on the sliding seat and rails.

It was amazing to get up so early, see the dawn, and be outside on the water at sunrise. I loved it. I have been told I'm the "I wanna do that" girl. I want to experience all the things. I want to see what it's like. Rowing crew was like that. I wanted to do that, and I did it. I didn't make any long-lasting friendships. I was quiet, kept to myself, put my head down, and did the work. It felt similar to being in the Civil Air Patrol.

I was the biggest girl on the crew team, so I knew I had to pull my weight. The total mass in the boat was important to keep down; if you were heavy, your contribution mattered even more. As a team, we did strength training in the winter and used the rowing machines in the armory's basement. We had 2,000-meter competition rows and relays. The coach was surprised at my strength and seemed satisfied that I contributed to the team. I could keep up on the rowing machines with the big guys, so he never cut me. We would jog outside on the trails and run stairs inside the CII (Center for Industrial Innovation) building. I was always the slowest and would have mixed feelings at the end of practice. I felt accomplished, and my endorphins were pumping, but I also felt bad about myself for always being the fattest and slowest.

Amanda failed out of RPI, so I continued into my sophomore year on the crew team without her. Practice was early, and everyone was always tired as hell, standing outside in the cold and getting ready to work out hard. The coxswain in the boat's bow ran the workout and inspired us to work harder or go slower or faster. There was one architecture student coxswain who was my favorite. He would sing R.E.M.'s song "Everybody Hurts," knowing we were all in pain from rowing so hard.

In the summer between first and second year, I found a crew team in Buffalo to join and rowed on the Niagara River in downtown Buffalo. I went to a meet in Syracuse and got to row on the toxic Lake Onondaga. The time I spent rowing crew led me to race in the Head of the Charles Regatta in Boston with many elite Ivy League schools. It was a privilege, and this was the first team sport I ever participated in that I felt a part of. I mean, I played softball in grammar school, but I never really felt like an athlete or a part of a team there. I was going through the motions. It was the same thing with tennis in high school and the rifle team; it was not really about being an athlete.

In the mornings after crew during freshman year, we would return, eat breakfast, and frequently go back to bed. I didn't have many 8 a.m. classes, and the ones I did were easy, so I could skip them. The school work freshman year was nearly a repeat of senior year of high school. Physics was easy. Math was easy. Intro to Engineering Analysis was easy. But in that class, attendance in the working groups was required.

They forced us into a team of four, and I got stuck with three boys. The first day, I was bright-eyed and asked them which problem they wanted to work on. They looked down and ignored me. So, I put my head down and worked on my problems. Occasionally, they would talk to each other, but none of them spoke to me or even made eye contact. After the first test was returned and I put my one hundred percent down on the table, they were all in shock. The next week, we showed up and started working, and one guy finally broke down and asked how I was doing one problem. So I started helping him, and this finally broke through the barrier.

This was a lesson I learned and took to heart for the rest of my career. Prove yourself. Put your head down, do the work, and people will come to you. It sucks that they wouldn't talk to me from the beginning. It sucks that my feelings were hurt. It sucks that as a female in STEM, you have to prove yourself, but that's the way things are.

This wasn't the only, nor the first time, that I was ignored as a female in engineering. The following year, in Intro to Engineering Design, we had a design and build project. We were in teams of five or six people, and again, I struggled to get people to talk to me. Eventually, after going to the machine shop and machining parts, they acknowledged me. We had to take the motor from a portable battery-operated screwdriver and a capacitor, which had a liquid center that changed capacitance based on angle, and use them to make a pipe inspecting gadget to measure the pitch of a pipe. We used the motor and a long worm gear in a two-piece design with articulating brakes. I designed and manufactured the motor mount and the gears and machined and fabricated the brakes. Two others built the housing out of composite; the last two guys did the electronics and programming. The two electronics folks took way too long, and we scrambled up until the last minute, pulling an all-nighter. It was stressful waiting and watching them, not knowing if we'd ever finish, and feeling powerless to help.

My social life began to click into place as well. Amanda, who was also the girl who was dating two men, turned out to be pretty toxic. However, her roommate Vanessa, a nuclear engineering student and one of the only girls who brought her own computer, ended up being a close friend of mine. We were also close to Kay, who was super involved in the Formula One racing team. Kay had a room full of go-kart racing trophies and was in the mechanical engineering program. We were all down-to-earth, normal, non-toxic, pitch-playing, pool-playing, nerdy science girls. Girls who you could trust and talk to; girls with whom you could play cards, play video games, read books, and share technology interests. I found my people.

Vanessa, Kay, and I got an apartment together on 15th Street. Our landlord loved and appreciated us because we always paid on time, cleaned, painted, built bookshelves, and many other things. If we painted anything, he would buy us a case of beer. We rarely called him in the three years we lived there, once when the boys who lived above us left the shower running, and it leaked, and once when the soap dish came off the wall in the shower. None of us had it in us to fix that because it needed to be re-drywalled and tiled and should be waterproof. He was so impressed by our practical nature. He said some of these RPI kids were really dumb, and one kid called him to ask if he could heat up the metal desk. Kay made curtains, and we painted the porch, the walls, and the trim in the living and dining rooms. The following summer, I painted and re-carpeted my bedroom.

The apartment was a long walk from campus, but we were okay with that. During freshman year, I did not have a car, but I eventually did and was grateful for it when the winter came. We learned to cook, and we occasionally had parties. The apartment was furnished, and we made the best of the place despite the brown indoor/outdoor carpet in the living and dining room.

We had an antenna TV with three channels. I remember one Saturday coming home from the library, making lunch, and sitting down to watch TV. Some race was on, and I was mesmerized. It turned out it was the 1995 Ironman triathlon race—140.6 miles. You swim 2.4 miles in the waves of the Pacific Ocean. Then you hop on your road bike, clip in your shoes (something I had never heard of), and bike for 112 miles. Then, after all that, you run a full marathon of 26.2 miles. All for a total of 140.6 miles.

This race was the year the female leader, Paula Newbie Frasier, bonked one mile from the finish. Her muscles all locked up, and she fell to the ground, sat on the curb, and nearly passed out. It was also the year that Mark Allen won at age thirty-seven, which was unheard of to win at that age. He also broke his record.

No bell went off in my head, nothing that screamed, *I wanna do that!* I didn't think about it much after it was over, but the seed was planted and must have percolated because in 2014, the words came out of my mouth without me consciously thinking about it.

I want to do an Ironman.

Motivational speaker Les Brown says, "Your dream was given to you." And I felt like that. It was like I was receiving a future already chosen for me.

Fine Lines

Obsession
like Elon Musk with the door handles
and
Howard Hughes with the rivets
I am obsessed with fine lines
SMOOTH
smooth curves
smooth figures
like the B-2 or F-14 wing
no cellulite
muscles defined
no jagged edges
no cumulus clouds
and the boundary between black and white
Fifty shades of
where is the line?
of worry, doubt, and paranoid
worry and OCD
check the lock? Nah
Fine Lines
I straddle, I find
food obsession
weigh and measure
binge and healthy
poor or rich
life or choice

red or blue
defensive or needy
angry or sad
right or wrong
Fine Lines
Oh how beautiful
smooth
fine lines we all look for
but are forever eluded

CHAPTER 23

Flying High

If they don't give you a seat at the table, bring a folding chair.

–SHIRLEY CHISHOLM

In 1996, I went on a co-op in Greenville, Texas, at a division of the Raytheon Corporation. A co-op was an entire summer and one semester working in the real world while still in undergraduate studies. Co-ops are mandatory at some schools, like Rochester Institute of Technology, but they were optional for RPI. I went anyway, figuring it would be good for my resume.

My mom helped drive me down there and then flew home. I got a 400-square-foot, one-room apartment with a kitchen with an eat-in bar countertop attached to one big room, a closet, and a bathroom. It had a futon for a bed, and that was it. No other furniture or TV or anything.

The first night, we sprayed Raid around the perimeter of the apartment, and the next morning, there were thousands of dead cockroaches everywhere. My mom even had them in her suitcase when she got home. We ended up calling Orkin and getting monthly service, which worked, thank goodness. It was by no means a palace, but it was mine.

In hindsight, it was universal foreshadowing that I started my aerospace career at Raytheon, my first official aerospace employer, and that I currently and likely will end my career working for Raytheon. I was excited, mostly nervous, and I hoped I could do this real-world engineering thing.

This particular site of Raytheon was as large as a university campus, with golf carts buzzing by as you walked from building to building. Texas heat was no joke, and having a windshield reflector was a must. On my first day looking out at the parking lot, I remember thinking how cool the sea of reflectors looked, and then I thought it's too bad they weren't solar panels.

This site had its own runway, with C-130s, C-5s, and KC-135s landing frequently. It was basically an avionics upgrade facility. Air Force One and the Royal Saudi Air Force both landed there when I was onsite. The aircraft would land, spend time in the hangars for upgrades (maybe up to a week), and then depart. The word would make it around if anything cool was in the hangar, and we could go see. When the Royal Saudi Air Force was there, it was guarded by men with assault rifles, probably every fifteen feet.

I worked in a building that seemed to be as far away from the runway as possible, with no windows. Once you got in, it was a boring tan cube farm. I worked on Computer-Aided Design (CAD), first learning on Unigraphics Ten, which had a space ball for a mouse. Some of the engineering changes I worked on included rearranging the cockpit avionics boxes and designing racks and mounts.

I finished all the work for my department and got lent out to another department with only a prior revision of Unigraphics, version nine, with a button box for commands. I felt like I jumped back to 1985. I was in charge of converting all 2D drawings to 3D models. The work was mindless, and I got adept at modeling and creating drawings swiftly. I remember we had to put in a 3D-modeled ninety-fifth-percentile man in some of the aircraft models. Most people don't know, but all airline seats are designed to fit the ninety-fifth-percentile military male. I kept looking at it, thinking, *This is NOT big enough for the average American.*

Work was fun, but the culture was more interesting. I was in an office with mostly white men who treated me well. I was never discriminated against or excluded, and I made friends to play cards with at lunch. I was surprised that they all fit the stereotype and wore cowboy boots and hats to work every day. I was complimented on my work and given more and more responsibility. I remember there was a fresh-out-of-college graduate who started the same time I did, and I helped him quite a bit. He also wore cowboy boots and hats, and when he heard the song "One Is the Loneliest Number" on the music that played all day on a low volume, he thought that was the weirdest song. It was like these people were stuck in a Texas airlock with no exposure to the rest of the world.

Raytheon had a flying club, and I decided that I wanted to train to be a private pilot. I went flying as much as I could. With the extra income and extra time, I could afford it. I loved it. I was nervous on my first solo flight. I kept telling myself to pretend my instructor was still in the aircraft, and I made a few loops while he stood on the side of the runway. Then we did night flying and "cross country" flights (longer than 300 nautical miles). I scheduled my final test in December, but it was canceled due to weather. I scheduled it two more times, and they were canceled too. I had to depart Texas and return to New York, and my disappointment was deep. I never finished my private pilot's license, but I'm proud and happy that I did as much as I could with my time in Texas.

Even though flying provided an outlet, I was immensely lonely when I arrived in Texas. I would go home from work, eat, and watch TV when I wasn't flying. I tried walking around and going to the mall, but honestly, I was a little afraid. I found out that there was a KKK rally in Greenville, and it made me nervous and self-conscious because of my brown skin. I felt like I was being watched and gawked at when I walked around outside. I ended up putting an ad in the Dallas paper in the personals for friends to show me around town.

I made one close friend I spoke to on the phone nearly every night. We only met in person twice for dinner, but it was nice to have someone to talk to. We were not attracted to each other, so having a best friend without the added pressure of a physical relationship was comforting. We argued about music, and he introduced me to Rush, a band I hadn't ever liked.

I bought an acoustic guitar and started to teach myself how to play with an *Easy Beatles with Tablature* book and a battery-operated tuner. One of the men who answered the ad also played guitar, and we met up a few times to practice.

He had a ton of sheet music and lent it to me. By the end of the six-month co-op, I had his "Stairway to Heaven" and "Dust in the Wind" sheet music and could play it. He was very friendly and somewhat attractive. I remember wanting him to want me, but he never made a move, so we just stayed friends.

I also met and went out with one guy, and we got a tattoo. When we talked on the phone, he said he had been wanting to get one and asked if I'd like to go too. I said sure, and he picked me up in his truck with a six pack in the front seat between us. I had never drank and drove at the same time nor had I ever seen anyone else do that. I walked into the tattoo parlor with no plans. I didn't know what I wanted or where. I looked through the books and chose a teal rose. I liked the teal because it was unique, and teal-colored roses don't exist anywhere in real life. I decided to put it in my cleavage. I have no idea why. Maybe to feel sexy. Maybe to be near my heart. I never saw him after that (and I don't even remember his name), but I have the tattoo to remember the wild adventure. I have no regrets.

The last fellow I met, I really fell for. His name was Jason, and he worked at the Naval Air Station in Fort Worth. He was dark-skinned like me, with dark brown hair, brown eyes, and a military body. I was drooling from the moment I saw him. We had a wonderful dinner at Rainforest Cafe, trying alligator for the first time. We drank wine and talked for what seemed like hours. We talked about airplanes, food, and music. He was a tech in charge of washing F-15s and F-16s, and he also said he thought these aircraft were so beautiful. I looked into his eyes, and we kissed right there. We ended up nearly ninety miles away, back at my place, and I took him to bed.

He had a tattoo on his shoulder that said "OHIO" in big, bold, black letters. I asked him about it the next day while we were still naked, laying in bed after five rounds of sex and having called off work. He said he was from Ohio, and getting the tattoo felt right. It's funny how I ended up in Cleveland years later. It's weird how you can only see those signs in hindsight.

He lived far away, and the phone conversation wasn't the greatest, so we ended up never seeing each other again. He said the phone calls felt like an obligation. I was hurt and sad but moved on quickly. It was no surprise that men didn't want me. It was a common occurrence, and I assumed it was always because of my weight.

I understand you don't want to be with a fat girl, I said to him in my mind. *Of course. Who does? Totally understandable. It's better than just being ugly, or bossy, or stupid, or boring I guess.*

See, Joyel? Everyone hates you.

CHAPTER 24

Grad School

You cannot build a better world without improving the individuals.

—MARIE CURIE

I went back to RPI having gained thirty pounds in Texas. Not being active. Not walking to class. Eating fast food or Chinese food nearly every night. I came back to Vanessa having found a man. Kay was good. The cats were fine. But everything seemed weird when I returned.

Kay and Vanessa only had one more semester, and now I had to stay for a full year. Vanessa's boyfriend didn't take a liking to me, and honestly, I felt like he stole my best friend, so I probably was pretty rude to him. My footing felt uneven, and I wanted the last semester to end and this to be over with. I was uncomfortable in my skin and new weight and therefore miserable.

I joined the RPI flying club with the intention of finishing my private pilot's license and went on several trips with them. This was pre-9/11, so we could fly lower than the New York City skyline. We flew between the towers of the George Washington Bridge. We took a trip to Portland, Maine for lobster dinner and then flew back. There was one scary landing at the airport in Albany, New York, where one of the students was training to get their IFR (instrument rating where you can fly in the clouds and rely only on your instruments), and it was super foggy that day. He was very nervous about landing, but we made it.

I started working in the RPI aero lab, which was in the basement of the Rickets building. I stumbled into this lab upon the suggestion of the administrative assistant of the mechanical and aeronautical department office. She told me to see Dan, the PhD student who ran the lab. When I went down to meet him, Dan was sitting at a desk with a computer and was so focused that he let me stand there for several minutes before he acknowledged me. I stood there and waited. When he was finally done with whatever he was concentrating on, he looked at me and asked if he could help me. I told him I was an undergrad looking for work.

Dan was nearly thirty and still running the lab as a PhD student, but he held a postdoc type of position. Since he had been there so long, he probably had about twenty experiments worth of research thesis material. He was funded by Dr. Leik Myrabo and Dr. Henry Nagamatsu's aeronautical research, mostly from NASA and a few other outside contracts, such as Lockheed Martin.

This lab was amazing. It had a four-by-six-foot test section enclosed wind tunnel, a one-by-two-foot test section enclosed wind tunnel, a shock tube, a hypersonic shock tunnel, a water tunnel, and a transonic blowdown tunnel. I had worked on my resume and had a copy with me. Dan asked if I had one and was impressed when I pulled it out of my pack. He hired me on the spot.

I began working there immediately for ten hours per week. I built an electrical box and bought a power supply with variable voltage and amperage. Dan had been looking for one for weeks, and my persistent efforts of calling every electrical, electronics, and electronics supply place in the phone book paid off. I found exactly what he was looking for, and he was super happy.

The lab was well stocked with anything you needed, and right down the hall was an old machine shop with a manual lathe, mill, band saw, drill press, grinder, and about 5,000 shelves of stuff. Any connector, bit, tooltip, or tool you needed was all on hand. A tall, heavy-set, older, bald man with suspenders named Charley ran the machine shop. Another undergrad student, Andy, started working there too. I learned how to calibrate load cells, how to program in LabVIEW, and how to input the calibration of the piezo electronic pressure sensor data into LabVIEW. Eventually, this work-study job landed me a paid internship and then fully funded grad school work on two NASA contracts in the hypersonic shock tunnel.

When I got back from co-op, I was off schedule from my previous classes, and many of my senior-year electives were taken with the junior class. I met a boy named George, who was a year younger and also an aeronautical engineer. He was in nearly all of my classes. He was tall and lean, with blond hair and blue eyes, perfect teeth, creamy skin. He was a nerd with a 4.0 average and super dorky. He was Ken!

But I definitely was not Barbie.

We had fun joking around in class and eventually started dating. He was in my Experimental Fluids class where we did experiments in the lab where I worked. We spent a lot of time clowning around the lab and looking at the other experiments I was working on. We went to lunch together, played racquetball, did homework together, and spent nearly every minute of his senior year together.

I was painfully aware that he did not like my weight. He never actually said anything to me, but I could tell by the way he flinched when he touched my belly fat. I began compulsively working out and started to drop weight, and I did what he said. I remember being at the pub with Andy and Dan, saying I needed to go home, shower, brush my teeth, and get ready to see George, and Andy commented that I should be able to be myself with him. Why was I doing all of this for a guy?

I brought George home for Thanksgiving. I was nervous and excited. I thought he was the one. When my cousin, four years younger and very attractive, came in the door, he was all over her, flirting like I had never seen him flirt.

Later that night, while we were lying in my twin bed holding each other, George whispered to me, "Your cousin is super cute."

"Get out of my bed!" I demanded.

He was startled and confused. I didn't know what else to say. Maybe in hindsight, I should have thanked him for his honesty. Perhaps I should have been sarcastic and said, "No shit, Sherlock." Either way, I was hurt.

I should have known then that he wasn't attracted to me. This was an Eckhart Tolle "pain body" scab that keeps getting ripped open. I couldn't believe it, but I also knew deep down that he never really wanted me. I was there for convenience. I was fun. I was a time killer. I was better than being alone.

I chose to keep dating him, knowing it was killing my soul. I secretly hoped I would win him over. I wanted him to be the one. I fantasized about our life together. We dated for the rest of the year, and I still had hope. I pined over him. I spoiled him. We went to New York City and saw *Phantom of the Opera*. We went to Massachusetts to visit his friend who wrote and performed a score for his school's orchestra.

When the time came, and he graduated, went off to work at Boeing, and I stayed back at grad school at RPI, I thought we would have a long-distance relationship. But it wasn't one month later that he broke up with me on the phone. I burned his photos, then had them re-developed from the negatives, and burned them again. I would cry in my room and stare at the pictures. I was not in my power. I gave it all away to him. I didn't care that he had all the power. I ignored my intuition and paid the price for that. Taking responsibility for your life means listening to that intuition.

CHAPTER 25

Self-Afflicting Hypocrisy

Change happens by listening and then starting a dialogue with the people who are doing something you don't believe is right.

—JANE GOODALL

When Kay and Vanessa graduated, I needed to find a place to stay. I found a house with three other grad students who turned out to be so much fun to live with. They cooked, watched *South Park*, and made smart, witty jokes.

During this summer, I went to my friend's house in Boston to see a free Barenaked Ladies concert, and she lent me Tony Robbins' *Personal Power* cassette tapes. This was the first time I ever listened to self-help books or tapes. I remember listening to them nonstop at my desk, taking notes. The key takeaway was that I own my power, mind, and story. He gave the example of people who have been victims of horrible pasts and said to play the story over with a different ending, putting colors and ice cream on it to heal the past. This did not work for me then, but it was an important first seed planted and later watered and sowed. I was blind at this age to the healing I might need to do. I had no idea what was beneath the layers of insecurity, loneliness, and low self-esteem.

In grad school, I had barely any classes. I got to play in the aero lab all day and typically ended the day at the RPI Union Pub, which had Newcastle and Bass beer on tap and was usually quiet. It was heaven, and life seemed easy and fun.

One day, Dan was trying to teach me something about fundamental quantum mechanics and what happens to the molecules in the hypersonic shock tunnel. He stood at the chalkboard and asked me questions. I would attempt to answer, and he would correct me.

Later that day at the pub, Dan said, "You're really defensive."

I was taken aback and shocked, and I realized that if I said anything, I would prove him right (self-afflicting hypocrisy). So, I found a response.

"In what way?"

"Well, when I try to teach you something, you get defensive."

"Ok, I see what you mean."

I sat and reflected on this a bit and then explained what I thought was happening.

"I think I want you to hear my line of thinking so you can tell me exactly where I went wrong. Or that I knew some of it and not all of it. And basically, I want you to think I'm smart."

"I do think you're smart. So stop doing that; it's annoying."

We laughed, and that was the end of it.

I tell this story often, especially when I see others or the people working for me do it. I think it's common not to want to be wrong. It's an ego protection. It's a story I've learned a lot from, and I still work on it. Many years after this first run-in with Dan, I was told by a CrossFit coach that I was not coachable.

"What?" I was taken aback.

"Next time you say '*I know*,' you're going to do a hundred push-ups," they barked back.

Crap. Ok.

I didn't realize I was doing it again.

I've hired a thousand coaches, and if any of them are reading this, they're probably like, *here it comes*. I have a bad habit of hiring coaches and not following their advice. Resistance.

What is going on with me? Besides the generic "the ego is getting in the way" answer, I found out what might be going on when I read Brianna Wiest's *The Mountain Is You*. I realized I constantly seek help from others, and when I get that coaching, I reject it.

She said we often seek what we actually need from ourselves, which almost appears to be the opposite of what we truly need. I realized that when I'm defensive or uncoachable, what I really need is to get quiet, seek, and listen to my own intuition. I don't need to be unteachable and reject others' opinions. I need to take in all the data, digest it, and determine what's right for me.

What I'm seeking from those teachers and coaches is validation, but what I need is to validate myself in my own choices and come into my own power—the babe with the power, you could say.

CHAPTER 26

Brent

Men often ask me, 'Why are your female characters so paranoid?'
It's not paranoia. It's recognition of their situation.

−MARGARET ATWOOD

It was my last semester at grad school. I still needed to get a full-time job lined up, but I knew it would happen soon. George was gone. Dan and Andy in the aero lab were my only friends.

One random day, I had a late-night class, and I thought I'd stop at the bar next to my apartment for a quick dinner and a beer. I sat on a bar stool in the dark, dingy bar and ordered wings and a beer. The man sitting next to me looked like a local, even though he was young. He started to talk to me, and I could tell I was right. I rolled my eyes internally. He was better looking than most locals, though a little grubby. He was a chatterbox. He told me his name was Brent, and he worked putting lawnmowers together at the Troy-Bilt factory. He talked about his ex-wife and his son and showed me the tattoo he had gotten for him. He said I was a pretty girl. I blushed.

Why are we, as women, so easy to get with those little words, "You're beautiful?" Is it only me? Is it only the women who never hear it? Or never get hit on? I think about my niece, who is drop-dead gorgeous. I assume she

120

hears it all the time, but maybe not. Maybe people figure she knows, so they never say it to her.

I never felt beautiful as a kid. I never said to myself, "Oh, I look cute," or "I like how I look in this outfit." I only felt like I looked fat, frumpy, and like a slob, and then I succumbed to looking that way. I gave up.

So when this chatty guy in the bar called me pretty, I ate it up. It didn't hurt that he was, well, pretty freaking hot. He was not the sharpest knife in the drawer, but he got through life on his looks, brute force, and persistence. He was *very* persistent.

I invited him back to my apartment and took him to bed. The next day, he came over, and we had sex again.

The next day, he said, "Let's go for a walk and out for beers." And then we did it again.

I overlooked all of his flaws, his dirty fingernails. Ironic that I judged him for being dirty when I never wanted to be judged for that as a child. I overlooked his poor, Brooklyn, broken English. I overlooked that he always smelled like cigarettes and his teeth were not very nice. I was embarrassed to introduce him to my other college friends, so I didn't. After a while, I felt like the relationship had run its course, but he kept coming over. He was the only boy who had ever kept coming back.

My phone would ring, and it would be him. "What are you up to?" he'd say.

"Homework."

"Ok, I'll be right over."

I'd complain to my roommate, "What the heck? He just comes over! I didn't invite him."

But then we'd have sex, and he'd leave.

My roommate and I would talk about Brent and how he was always super cocky, trying to show off and joke around when he met people. One day, he came over, and we watched the Yankees game. He was calm, kind of chill.

"Today, he wasn't that bad. I kind of enjoyed hanging out with him today," my roommate admitted.

And my mind and perspective changed. I thought maybe I could be with him. When the cocky SOB wore off, what was deep down, what was left, was okay. What I didn't know was the cocky SOB came back with a vengeance when he was drunk and horny.

We played the computer game *You Don't Know Jack* and drank and had sex and watched Yankees games and had more sex. Then, it came time for me to graduate. I got a job in Ohio working at NASA Glenn Research Center. I stressed about what to do with Brent. I didn't seek advice. I didn't ask or talk to anyone. It just came out of my mouth one day in the car.

"Do you want to go with me?"

He quit his job at Troy-Bilt and moved out with me.

Part of what attracted me to Brent was that he was a real bad boy. It excited me to be on the arm of a former Brooklyn guy who hung out with mobster brothers, sold drugs in Washington Square Park, had been arrested on more than one occasion, and did who-knows-what-else. His stories were vague but exciting. I badly wanted him to buy that 1980s black leather jacket and wear a white T-shirt. I never asked, but he probably would have.

We had fun, fantastic sex, and he looked up to me. He bragged to his family that he was dating a rocket scientist.

His sister would laugh and say, "It took a rocket scientist to figure out my brother."

He admired my intelligence. He trusted me. He gave me confidence in bed, and the many times I would get jealous or feel fat or disgusting, he made me put my hands over my body and told me I was beautiful.

"Feel this. This is beautiful," he'd say.

I didn't listen. I didn't let it fully sink in because the pain was too deep. But he appeased me momentarily, and I could be free and happy with him. I could walk around the house naked and feel like a million bucks. The whole time we were in New York, we never fought.

I had no idea what was to come.

Fuck Me

Fuck Me
Make me whole
Need Me
Make me important
Praise Me
Make me proud
Smile at Me
Make me smile back
Hug Me
Make me loved
Protect Me
Make me safe
Talk to Me
Make me interesting
Cook for Me
Make me full
Caress Me
Make me loved

PART 4

Under Jareth's Spell

CHAPTER 27

NASA

I've been in so many spaces where I'm the first and only
Black trans woman or trans woman period. I just want to work
until there are fewer and fewer 'first and only's.'

−RAQUEL WILLIS

I started working at NASA in June of 1999, and it was like a dream come true. Driving up through those gates, the campus felt like a university. All the wind tunnels an aeronautical engineer could ever dream of. I was excited to be a part of this organization, with a wide variety of diverse men and women who had been through these gates. I was happy I wasn't an "only" or "first" girl in the room.

Although I had filled out many forms in my life where you have to check the box denoting race, I had never been blatantly asked, "How come you didn't check Hispanic?" This time, I was.

"I'm only half," I explained to the HR rep. "And I was raised with white privilege. I don't feel it's right or fair to check that box."

I felt like I would be taking away an opportunity from someone else. I thought it would be fraudulent because I wasn't raised Hispanic and couldn't even speak Spanish. The pure fact that I had to explain this to someone infuriated me. I knew they only wanted to improve or increase their diversity metrics. And while this might have been the first time this came up, it wasn't the last.

I was excited to work at NASA, but I wasn't super excited about my job title—Data Engineer. It sounded boring and simplistic. I was maintaining a long list of sensors (temperature, pressure, load cell, etc.) used to operate the Propulsion Systems Lab (PSL). This full-scale jet engine test facility simulated flying up to 90,000 feet with proper inlet air pressure and temperature. I maintained the list of sensors from the customers that were on the engine. I was in charge of calibrations and ranges of amps and volts.

In hindsight, this was an important job, and I was ignorant in my dislike for the job title. At the time, I thought it was beneath me. I thought I was capable of so much more. What I didn't know then was an important life lesson about putting in your time.

I worked with computer science folks to get the data acquisition system up and running for each test, inputting all of this data, importing customer engine performance code, and setting up screens for the control room. Ramp up and down for engine testing could be long, taking months of pre-work and setup for testing that we only ran for about a month at a time, two or three times a year. The actual engine testing was an adrenaline-filled, long-hours adventure. The control room for the test cell felt like a real Houston Mission Control and basically looked like that.

During testing, we'd have the engine manufacturers (our customers) in the control room request to change the data acquisition system screens ad hoc. Many sensors would go down and break, so we'd have to improvise on the fly. I wished I could run tests all year long. My work was my passion.

As exciting as the tests were, the government work stereotype was true at NASA. There were long periods of waiting. There were days when I drove down to the Metroparks and took a nap because work was so boring it made me want to sleep at my desk, and I didn't want to do that.

Brent moved with me to Cleveland, even though we had only been dating for a few months. Our apartment complex was in an upscale southern suburb of Cleveland with good schools and on the edge of being rural. We rented a two-bedroom, two-bath, new construction apartment that looked like a townhome on the second floor of a three-floor building. The apartment had a garage and a balcony. The complex had a pool, weight room, and a large venue you could rent for parties.

Brent tried to impress me and did the cooking and cleaning while looking for a job. Looking back, I failed early on in our relationship by constantly criticizing, condemning, and complaining. I hardly ever gave him any positive feedback for all his efforts. This, of course, made him stop trying so hard. It was a lesson I learned much later in life after taking the Dale Carnegie course and book *How to Win Friends and Influence People*. I realize now that I set him up to give up. If nothing is ever good enough, why bother?

I remember the day the movers came, and Brent set up the bookshelf and put plants on it. I grimaced and started fixing things. I never said "Thank you," "Nice job," or "It looks nice." I could see his instant disappointment. I could see his face, hopeful of praise (or positive feedback) and then instantly sad and let down. He checked out, flopped on the couch, and gave up.

I invited Brent to lunch with my boss the first week. I think Brent was nervous, and I was, too. It went okay, but I could tell my boss's feelings were the same as my family's. *You can do better, Joyel.* I don't actually know what anyone was thinking. Remember, my family never talks about real things. But my friends would be so blunt.

"What are you doing with him?" they'd say.

They planted seeds of doubt in our relationship, but I blatantly ignored them and my intuition. I knew, too. I knew from the first time he spoke to me in that bar, but I chose to ignore that little voice inside. He paid attention to me. He told me I was beautiful over and over again. He and his family constantly gave me praise I never got. They were talkers, unlike where I grew up. Nothing was left unsaid. It was all always out on the table.

I started to feel like my home life wasn't so great. All we did was drink and party. I hated cooking and doing all things domestic—laundry, cleaning. I wanted to go back to school, to be learning. Work was amazing in some ways, but super slow and kind of boring. I was depressed every day driving home. I didn't want to come home, even though I had a very nice, super clean, new apartment in North Royalton. Deep down, I knew I deserved better than Brent, but I didn't want to admit it and didn't know how to send him packing.

My weight was plaguing me also. Always. I didn't feel satisfied or comfortable in my skin. I knew I was with the wrong partner but didn't know how to get out of it. I was eating until I was comfortably numb. I was drinking too much on the weekends, making me hungover. I had no hobbies or projects. I was bored.

We went out drinking a lot. Most of the time, we would get tipsy, but occasionally, or maybe every Friday or Saturday, we would get way too drunk. Brent always wanted to have sex when he was drunk, and if I wasn't as wasted as he was, I would get annoyed and say no. And then he would get *really* angry. It was the same fight we would have for nearly the next seven years.

One ordinary night of partying, for some reason, we had a bottle of Wild Turkey bourbon that we had been drinking with coke. We went to bed a tiny bit more than buzzed, but not so drunk that we were stumbling around. I remember being happy, the giddy kind of happy. I had just gone off the pill, perhaps at the advice of a doctor or therapist, so we were using condoms. We had sex, and it was good. I don't remember the conversation afterwards, or how we started going again, but round two started up. We didn't have another condom, so we decided to use the same one (gross, I know). I was on top the first time, but Brent was on top the second time. And I swore I felt him come inside of me.

Even though we were both drunk, I remember feeling like, *OMG, I'm pretty sure we just made a baby.* (Flash of *Hot Tub Time Machine* "I feel pregnant.") And I was right. I wasn't scared or freaked out. I was surprisingly happy. It wasn't in my plan. I wasn't thinking about it or avoiding it. I was mindlessly going through life, and bam, baby! This magical feeling was for sure a Universal Sparkle, a flicker of light, like the Universe said, *This is why you're together.*

Even though I was twenty-four years old, with a job, and on my own, I was terrified to tell my mom. She was not a fan of Brent. I called her at work, hoping for a quick conversation. I was shocked to hear her joy on the other side of the line. She was thrilled. She said she loved babies and couldn't wait.

I was itching to get out of the apartment, so we started looking for a house. We found a nice small home on the west side of Cleveland on West 148th Street. It was perfect, and I still have fond memories of that little place. Unfortunately, it wasn't in the best school district, and I used to drive down to Strongsville and pine over the Bob Schmidt homes there. Eventually, we found one that was pretty run down on sale for much less than it was worth. An older couple wanted to be done with taking care of the house. We bought it and moved again a couple of years later. Little did I know the time in that beautiful Bob Schmidt home would be some of the hardest years of my life.

CHAPTER 28

Landmark

The thought beneath so slight a film
Is more distinctly seen

–EMILY DICKINSON

I can't remember who turned me onto Landmark or where I heard of it, but I attended a three-day retreat in a hotel conference room when I was pregnant in late 2000, right before Andrew was born in January 2001. It was similar to what I imagine an original Tony Robbins, smaller-sized, personal growth retreat would be like. There were maybe 250 people in attendance.

The leader would stand onstage and lecture for a while, asking probing questions. He would bring up a person and ask them why they were there. I didn't know why I was there. I was there to fix my unhappiness, my food issues, my overall negative mental disposition. Then, you'd have to break up into small groups or write alone for a while about a topic and then share something deeply personal with strangers. I loved the nature of this self-exploration, being transparent with myself and a stranger, pulling the Band-Aid off, and exposing the truth. For me, this was the start of the work—the true puzzle-solving of the labyrinth.

There was a woman who raised her hand in the beginning. "I can't sit all day

132

in these chairs, so I'm going to get up and walk around in the back occasionally."

"Okay." The leader approved and kept going.

Since I was seven months pregnant, I thought the same thing. I also sat in the back with her, and in the beginning, I also got up and stood or walked around a bit.

Landmark was a derivation of the Erhard Seminar Training (EST) system of the 1970s, which received bad publicity for making people stay in the conference without letting them out to use the restroom.

Spoiler alert: If you're ever interested in attending one of these seminars, I'm giving away the goods here.

The purpose of the whole three-day weekend retreat was for you to identify your story and your beliefs and come to realize that they are all bullshit, made up by you, and in your control to change. Landmark posits that life is empty and meaningless, and that's a good thing because you get to define the meaning for whatever end or purpose you decide.

Their point was that your mind, beliefs, and story control your body, future, and outcome. The seminar was the first time I'd heard about the mind's stream of thought and how it controls you. It was the first time I'd realized the power of the mind and the tapes I played repeatedly in mine.

One of the initial exercises was to sit still and think about your right hand. You pull all your energy into the right hand for sixty seconds, getting it warm and tingly. Then, you open your eyes and take your right hand into your left hand. I could feel the difference. The point of the exercise is to realize the power of your mind. Once you realize this and that this applies to everything, you begin to see that you can make yourself anxious or calm, all based on the stories you tell yourself.

My first thought was, *Can't I just think about working out and get my heart rate up and never have to actually work out?*

Well, maybe, but I think that would take a lot of mastery (another limiting belief, perhaps).

We spent time in this seminar writing our story out, re-writing it, and then reading it ten times until we realized it was bullshit. (Kind of similar to writing a memoir.) I chose to write about my weight and my food issues.

I read it to a strange man. He didn't understand. I didn't write thoroughly enough to get it all out, and the power of my issue wasn't exactly resolved in that seminar. But many seeds were planted.

After talking about our story, how our current interpretation might have been different from what happened, how we can change it, and how it impacts us, the big ah-ha for me was in the end. Life is inherently empty and meaningless, and all this shit that happened to me in my life, while factual, was neither good nor bad. I could assign any meaning I wanted to it. It either has a negative or positive impact on me. I can choose.

In the movie *Labyrinth*, Sarah uses red lipstick to mark arrows on the floor tiles to remind herself which paths she's already taken. But some pesky creatures keep popping up from under the tiles and turning the arrows in different directions. That was my brain. I was earnestly trying to learn lessons and mark my path, but my thoughts and beliefs were sabotaging me. Not anymore. Suddenly, I could transform the old belief that everyone hates me into something more empowering. I could tell myself, *I am a boss. And sometimes people don't like that, but I love it. And people will eventually fall in love with me and my leadership.*

What I found interesting was how I *believed* I could not sit in those chairs for long because I was seven months pregnant. I got up frequently and walked around. By the end of the three-day session, I sat without rising and was captivated. The story of me being stiff, needing to get up, and my back hurting was gone. The same thing happened to the other lady who said she could not sit for long. It occurred to me that the original EST seminar's intention to make people sit without being allowed to go to the bathroom was to prove their point.

The mind achieves what the mind believes.

While the outcome I wanted from this seminar was a perfect body and unending happiness, the results were far different. Instead, I solved another part of the labyrinth. I let down my guard a little at work. I realized I didn't really know anyone there and wanted to be more open and transparent.

Before Landmark, I kept to myself, guarded and quiet. The next day, I went to work and turned my desk to be more open to my officemates, who I barely spoke to. I started to ask about their kids and how their weekend was. I made friends with the girl who sat next to me. I traded her my guitar for a keyboard. I went to her house to see her sewing projects. I made friends with some people at the Propulsion Systems Lab (PSL) at NASA. I did yoga with one friend, had sushi for the first time with two coworkers, made jokes and talked about aircraft with others, and talked about beer at the American Institute of Aeronautics and Astronautics (AIAA) Ground Testing Technical Committee (GTTC) with my boss.

The rest of the Landmark seeds took a little more time to sow in my brain, but they eventually grew.

CHAPTER 29

Baby Blues

Birth is the epicenter of women's power.

–ANI DIFRANCO

I loved being pregnant. I felt healthy and like I was listening to my body for the first time. I searched for prenatal yoga classes and signed up for my first yoga class. It was wonderful, peaceful, and nurturing for my body. My mom's friend gave me all her maternity clothes, and I was super excited that they fit. She was "normal" size, and I was plus size. I was not expecting they would fit, but she was pregnant with twins, and most maternity clothes are pretty stretchy.

Andrew's birth was many hours of calm excitement followed by one hour of unstoppable pain. I was at work on a Friday and started to feel some cramps. A few weeks earlier, I had gone into the hospital for Braxton Hicks, so I figured that's all it was this time, too. It was still several days before Andrew's due date, and I thought we weren't ready yet. I decided after a while that they were getting pretty regular and that I better go to the hospital.

I went into the hospital on Friday around noon. I was already a little bit dilated, so they decided to keep me. I called Brent, my mom, and my two friends who were from RPI and also anxiously awaiting Andrew. He was born twenty-four hours later. Although we went to the Lamaze classes and I'd seen a bunch of movies depicting childbirth, I was not expecting what occurred. I was surprised by the instinctual cues. I felt like a dog who had the instinct to tamp a bed down and go around in circles. I was bossy (big surprise) and asked and advocated for what I needed.

I told the nurse I wanted to get naked.

"Go ahead."

I told the nurse I wanted to squat.

"Squatting is the best."

They let me do whatever I wanted.

My water didn't break until about an hour before, and once that happened, it seemed to go quickly. I asked for pain meds, and they said it was too late. I remember thinking that I needed a break, I needed it to stop, that I couldn't do this. I felt like I was running a marathon against my will. I remember thinking this would be much easier if I were in better physical shape. After a lot of pain and screaming and thrashing around, Andrew arrived at 12:04 pm on January 20 while George W. Bush was on the TV in the background being inaugurated.

I always knew I wanted to name my firstborn after my grandfather. Grandpa was my buddy, my spelling list study partner, my go-to for playing catch in the front yard, my bike ride companion, my dollhouse-making carpenter. He was the one who always gave me fifty dollars when I came home from RPI, who always gave me money for good report cards, and who unconditionally accepted me for who I was, dirty fingernails and all. Grandpa's name was Andrew H. Kerl, so my sweet little baby was also named Andrew.

When Andrew was born, my mom visited and stayed with us for two weeks. Our first house was a small, A-frame, 1,000-square-foot, three-bedroom, one-bath house near NASA on the west side of Cleveland. My mom went grocery shopping and bought a ton of food, including a bunch of junk food—sweet breads, cinnamon buns, and Entenmann's coffee cake. I was thinking to myself, *How much sugar, flour, and butter can we eat?* A lot.

I was crying all the time. She would criticize my crying, telling me this wasn't normal and that I should do something about it, but she would not be specific about what to do. I thought it was normal and would go away.

I was surprised that she didn't know how to take care of my son as much as I thought she would. I had envisioned her teaching me. Instead, she was hesitant and walked on eggshells around me, not wanting to actually help. My in-laws came out also, but they stayed at a hotel and were only there for about a day. They brought Brent's previous son with them. He was adorable with Andrew. My mom was uncomfortable around them and continued to bake and eat. She baked cakes and ate and fed them to me. It was not a good time.

My anxiety about breastfeeding kept me from fully releasing milk. I remember going back to the hospital to get help, and while the nurse was validating that I was doing it right, my milk finally let down. That was the first and last time it happened. When I returned home, I could never fully relax enough to let it happen. Andrew cried for what seemed like all the time, and the only thing that appeased him was trying to nurse. But he'd fall asleep and never actually get anything. After a couple of weeks of hell, I gave him a two-ounce bottle of formula, and he slept for four hours straight. I felt like a new woman. So, I gave up breastfeeding. I figured he got some good stuff, and I called it a day.

One of the early days when I was still home on maternity leave, Brent left and went to work or the store. Andrew was sitting in one of those bouncy seats on the kitchen table, and I spoke out loud to him.

"Look, man, it's just you and me. We're in this together." I stared at him, no smile on either of our faces.

I'm unsure why I felt this way or what projection I had about being a single mom. Brent was obviously not going anywhere at that point. But it felt like Andrew and I were tied at the hip, and for some reason, we were alone in the world together. I was pleading with him to get better and stop being so fussy because we were in this together forever.

I definitely did not feel what I think most new moms are supposed to feel. I didn't smile much at Andrew. I didn't love being a new mom. I was anxious and worried about doing it wrong. Andrew was not a particularly happy baby either. I would take him to the mall and walk around, and we would both be content for a few hours. But at home, it was bad vibes all the time.

All I wanted to do was sleep. Always. I couldn't wake up. I would get to work and want to go home and sleep. I would drop Andrew off at daycare, come home, and go to sleep. I would go to work and then go home sick to sleep. Or I would leave work, drive down the road to the Metroparks at lunch, and sleep. In hindsight, I had postpartum depression, but I kept thinking it would go away or get better within a few weeks.

It didn't.

I finally got help when the baby was eight months old. I started to see a therapist and was put on medication. One day, when I was sitting on the floor playing with Andrew in my living room, he turned his head. I looked at his cute little head, and I finally felt that overwhelming love for him. I was like, *Ohhhhh, this is what love is.*

But as big as the love finally was, I remember it tied very closely with fear and pain. I thought, *Oh my god, someone is going to hurt this kid someday. And I will bash their head in.*

It all came to me at once. All the love and all the pain. I wanted to squeeze him and protect him. I was excited about his life and couldn't wait to do all the cute and fun things with him. At the same time, my mind was screaming, *Please, please, please don't ever let him get hurt.*

What Do Strong Women Do in Times Like This?

You can't wash away your womanhood
In a hot shower.
You can't wash away past sex
In a hot shower.
You can't wash away the images
In a hot shower.
You can't wash away your boobs or your fat or your vagina
In a hot shower.
You can't wash away your womanhood
In a glass of wine
or hamburger
or the arms of your husband.
It might never go away.
You can feel all the feels
Stick with it
Find the words.
What do strong women do in times like this?
Spiral, look for the escape hatch.
Then sit.
Write the words.
Take the showers again.
Be present.
Do the next right thing.
Think of Sally McRae and what she's been through.
Chip away at the walls of the pain cave like Courtney DeWalter.

Strong women.
One foot in front of the other.

CHAPTER 30

Suicidal Tendencies

If you do not tell the truth about yourself, you cannot tell it about other people.

–VIRGINIA WOOLF

I didn't want to go home.

It was a sunny, cold winter day in Cleveland, and my mom picked me up from the airport. I wanted to see Andrew, but I didn't want to go home.

Thanks to my boss, I had just been to an AIAA conference where I was now a part of the Ground Testing Technical Committee (GTTC). It was a wonderful experience to go to the meetings, attend sessions where research was being presented, visit the large exhibit hall, and pick up a bunch of free swag from all the aerospace vendors. I got to sit with like-minded engineers working on setting the precedents and writing the procedures for future members to read. I joined a couple of committees on thrust stand and wind tunnel calibration since that was precisely what I was working on at NASA. I even took over the AIAA GTTC newsletter and published it for several years.

But after the escape of work, life was still waiting at home. Andrew was turning a year old in a week, and my mom and grandpa had come out to visit. I still hadn't fully recovered from postpartum depression. I didn't know if the meds hadn't kicked in or if it was the reality of returning to a life that I didn't think I wanted. I only knew I didn't want to go home.

Aside from postpartum depression, I was struggling at this time to decide whether or not to get Andrew baptized. I didn't want to, but I felt obligated. I didn't have the fight in me to stand up to my mother, and I knew I didn't want to disappoint my grandpa. So I decided that I'd go through the motions. If I was wrong about this no-God thing, then this was cheap insurance.

I found a Catholic church very close to my house on the west side of Cleveland. I called the priest and made an appointment to meet and talk about baptizing Andrew. I was honest about where I was with my agnostic, religion-hating state of being, and the priest was open to having these conversations. He agreed with one of the people I found in a science and religion magazine, Rabbi Rami, who said that all religions are good, that everything is God, and that religions are like languages used to speak to God. This priest also suggested that most people stick around for the ritual. People like ritual because there is something pure and honest about it.

I liked him, and he was willing to baptize my precious baby even though I would not attend church or ever go back there. I was grateful for his kindness, openness, and willingness to have these discussions with me. I felt validated in my own beliefs and skin.

Around this same time, Brent and I decided to get married. He never officially proposed, and I purchased my own wedding ring and even paid for the trip to the Bahamas to elope. The vacation was fun, but deep down, I knew this wasn't right, and I ate to cope with it.

The day I got married, I was the heaviest I had ever been. I weighed over 300 pounds. Wearing a plain, spaghetti-strap, stretchy, white dress, not fitted, standing on the beach, I married my son's father. Brent was happy. I was doing what I thought I should to fit the mold. Making my bed because I had laid in it. I remember saying my vows feeling like a fraud. But I did it for Andrew. I did it to comply with societal expectations. Even though I was screaming inside, I chose not to listen to that girl.

I went to work daily and came home to a house I knew I shouldn't be in, married to a man I shouldn't be married to. We didn't drink as much, but when I did, I didn't want Andrew to see me. I would sip wine on the front porch.

Brent would get drunk frequently with his work friends. Some days, he would get drunk enough that he would call me to come pick him up. One time, he was so drunk that I couldn't understand what bar he was in. I could make out the street, which was Lorraine Avenue. If you've ever been to Cleveland, you'd know Lorraine Avenue is long. I drove up and down that road looking for his car, continuously extending my length until I finally found him.

Brent and I fought and fought often. I can't remember what we were arguing about, but one time, I picked up a plastic child's toy table and threw it across the room. Andrew screamed. I scared him, and I scared myself. I cried and held him. The next time I went to therapy, I told her about this incident. I admitted that I might need to go to anger management because I was afraid of what I might do. She sent me, and the depression and anger were still there.

Two years later, I was still going to therapy. I had been on a roller coaster of different antidepressants. I struggled to work consistently. I got sick frequently. I wanted to be in bed.

It was at this point that suicidal ideation started quietly weaving itself between my thoughts. I considered how I might do it. I remembered the razors in the garage. I took baths and many times brought a razor with me. I would put it to my skin and attempt to cut myself. I was surprised at how hard I had to push to get even a little bit of blood. I thought about the times when I cut when I was younger. Slight cuts, and I'd bleed. But on the wrist, it took a lot more pressure to get a deep cut. I never had the guts to push harder, to go deeper with the razor blade. Or maybe I didn't really want to leave Andrew.

I think about this now and cannot believe I was that close. I can't believe I would have given up this life and Andrew. I thought he would be better without me. I thought Brent was doing a good enough job, and Andrew would be better with just him than with a miserable mom. These are lies a person with severe depression tells themselves. The mind can be a scary, odd place.

I went to work, and I was barely a mom at home. My RPI friend had moved away, and I had no close friends. I had people at work I would go to lunch with occasionally who I was friendly with, but I was not tight with anyone. I didn't have a close relationship with my mom at the time. I was pleasant enough with some neighbors, but nothing meaningful. I had no gym that I was going to. I wasn't cooking, barely cleaning.

I ended up voluntarily checking myself into a place to get better. I spent two weeks there, literally almost the entire time sleeping. Finally, near the end of my stay, they made me attend the group therapy sessions. I worked up enough courage to go and started to make progress. I was surprised by the number of "normal-looking" people there. It wasn't like the movie *Girl Interrupted*. It was simply filled with people who couldn't take real life for one more minute.

I got out and went to group therapy twice a week. No one at work knew. My mom didn't come to visit. I felt very alone. Brent was just trying to manage. I learned in the depression workshop about planned pleasant activities (something to look forward to). I learned the importance of sleep, daily regulated caffeine intake (keep it the same each day, not too much, a little is good), and managing my food, alcohol, water, and exercise. It wasn't just to be physically healthy in a bodily way; it was necessary for brain chemistry to keep me alive. With that workshop and the combination of continued therapy and medication, I climbed slowly out of the woods.

I can now look back on that time and clearly and resolutely say, *Get. To. Therapy.* If you have an inkling you need it, then you need it. I waited way, way, way too long. I knew something was wrong, and I chose to ignore it. I didn't get it taken care of, and I almost lost this beautiful life.

I had to learn that I needed help to see a paradigm shift. I needed help to learn to take personal responsibility for my life. I realized that blaming others, God, life, or the Universe for my situation won't get me anywhere. I learned that feeling helpless is a victim mentality and that standing on my own two feet and not blaming the world for my situation is better than feeling like a victim of happenstance.

I needed to take control, and that meant getting help.

CHAPTER 31

A Crack in the Door

Your own personal Jesus

—DEPECHE MODE

Therapy and medication started to take hold, and the gray fog of depression began to lift. I could see the house now, and I wanted to make it more beautiful—painting, gardening, cooking, and making positive changes. I started working out a little at the NASA Glenn Fitness Center. Andrew got into the NASA daycare, the most wholesome daycare center I've ever seen. There were hot food lunches and age-appropriate playgrounds for each group.

The one constant, nagging issue was that I was still struggling with my weight, and it seemed to be the thing that commanded my mood and attention at all times. I joined Weight Watchers for about the fifth time. I was in a meeting and remember saying, "I just can't stick to my points for like one single day." The lady just looked at me. No comment, no advice. She just stared. She didn't know what to say. She had no words of encouragement. She made me feel like I was a strange outlier.

I would compulsively consume self-help books and found my way to Geneen Roth. She promotes "The Eating Guidelines," and I couldn't follow those either. In one of her books, she mentioned Overeaters Anonymous

(OA). I looked up where I could go to a meeting and attended my first one.

It was one of the more intimate meetings around Cleveland. It was in a small westside church, with only about four other people at the table. Everyone seemed awkward. I was grateful for a young, healthy-looking girl sitting next to me. The other members were much older and very quiet.

They all went around the table at the end of the meeting, and I didn't know what to say. I started crying. I ran out of the room, and the young girl followed me. It was winter, and we got stuck outside. I was and am so grateful she followed me and stood and talked with me in the cold for those ten minutes. I started attending meetings, and it was the first time I ever felt people were talking about something real. They call it sharing their "experience, strength, and hope."

I was excited to hear the stories and hopeful that I would recover enough someday to share my stories. I was eager to work the steps and clean out all the rubbish of guilt and shame I was carrying around. I thought back to the priest who baptized Andrew, who said to me, "You know, it doesn't have to be like this. You can have a spiritual connection without going to church or believing anything from the Catholic religion."

OA opened the door back up to having some sort of connection to a higher power. One of the steps is to accept a higher power and turn your life over to that higher power. Of course, being an atheist at the time, I squirmed in my seat and rolled my eyes. I did not want to surrender to anything. I would listen to others who struggled with the definition of higher power, too, and some would choose Mickey Mouse or some other thing or inanimate object as their higher power. *That's odd*, I thought, and I kept listening.

One day, I considered the weather. Water and the weather are certainly a higher power than myself. I can and do surrender every day to whatever the weather is. The great forces of nature like gravity, nuclear, and electromagnetism are certainly more powerful than I. There's an army of microbes and viruses that can kill me. And I remembered Rabbi Rami's German saying, "Alles ist Gott," which translates to "Everything is God." He states each religion is simply the language to speak to God. We choose what religion we want that we are most familiar with.

I started to consider that maybe, just maybe, these were all just words. They could mean whatever I wanted them to mean.

So, I looked up at the moon and said, "Hi God?"

Like I was seeing if that fit. Could I call the moon God? Maybe, yeah, I could try that on, like trying on a sweater. It kind of fits.

I would look at the trees and say, "Hi, God," and accept that nature and how we describe the natural world (science) would be the language I chose to speak to God.

The Universe is God. It is what it is. For me, it's described in math, physics, and chemistry. It IS God. It's all God. The languages of Catholicism, Christianity, Judaism, Hinduism, or Islam do not make sense to me because they are not the language I speak. That doesn't mean it's not right. I don't have to speak or learn any other language, or I can. It makes no difference.

Having this tiny bit of compartmentalizing God in a way that I could understand felt like finally organizing the linen closet efficiently. It felt like finally things made sense. The more I thought about it, the more it clicked into place. The molecules I breathe and exchange with the Universe and the fact that we're all just made of stardust make me feel at peace. This settled something in me and put angst to rest.

One puzzle solved. One million more to go.

CHAPTER 32

Outside Medicine

The only person you are destined to become is the person you decide to be.

–RALPH WALDO EMERSON

After I let the door crack a little and let the people from OA in a bit, I started to feel happy. I started to believe in what these wonderful people told me—that I was worthy of love, that they loved me. I believed them when they said they would love me until I learned to love myself. I would sit on their couches, have parties, and go to dinner every Monday night at Diana's in Lakewood. I would have the deepest conversations about loving my thighs. These beautiful, strong, God-given thighs to *me*. MY thighs.

One of the girls in OA that I hung out with a fair bit got me outside more. We went hiking, kayaking, camping, and built sweat lodges with her dad. She babysat Andrew, and she brought me back to nature.

Cleveland has this glorious park nicknamed the Emerald Necklace. It's this skinny swath of land that starts at the top of the lake and goes all the way around the city of Cleveland, forming a necklace of foliage around the city. Considering I lived and worked on the west side, I spent most of my time there—bike riding, sleeping in a parked car at lunchtime, taking walks, and choosing the long way home just to drive through the park.

I remember one fall day picking Andrew up from NASA daycare. I was driving home and decided to go to the Metroparks and take him for a little walk. We parked and began walking, and I was overwhelmed with awe and the smell of the fall air. The scenery wasn't any different than the day prior. Today wasn't particularly good or bad. But something was different in me. I was flooded with an appreciation for the nature around me in the same way that the love of my child had washed over me. It was love. It was contentment. It was healing. It was all of it wrapped up in a bow.

This was the moment I learned to trust the instinct. To me, the instinct was that little voice that said to stop in the park that day. I don't know why I stopped on this particular day. How many times had I ignored that voice? Countless. How many times had I ignored this path? Countless. How many times will I make the same mistakes and follow the love of Jareth? The answers were right there, outside, accessible to me always.

My mood immediately improved so drastically and noticeably that I wanted more of it. Of course, plenty of research shows the improved mood of being outdoors, especially if you go out more than forty-five minutes daily. I didn't realize or think of it, but when I started at NASA right out of college, I went from walking around campus daily outside to almost no outdoor physical activity.

After this realization, I made it a point to buy a mountain bike and to walk, bike, hike, or kayak as much as possible. I had no real physical goals at this time, but I knew I felt free and like a kid on the bike. I attended the NASA gym, worked with their trainers, and occasionally ran outside, but my physical fitness was still very poor.

It was this specific moment in time that was pivotal for me to realize how much I loved being outside—not just sitting on the porch stargazing but actually moving around, putting my hands in the soil. I am happy I found this external antidote to my internal battles, but of course, I had to learn this lesson many times over. I still had many future dark periods in my life where I didn't prioritize myself or my outdoor medicine.

Carry Me Out

How many times?
He is dead and he is dying
Spend your life soul searching
for a soul that died years ago
Don't bother going out on a limb
                        there's no fruit left
Crawl back within
Savour what is left of your thoughts
                        think and think
Until you stop shaking
And your blood stops
boiling, your brow starts
drying and then
relax and smoke a cigarette, but
                        stay squatting
always aware
don't let your guard down
'cause he'll always be there

CHAPTER 33

Just Keep Swimming

Fall down seven times, stand up eight.

—JAPANESE PROVERB

After a year in OA, I broke my "abstinence." It's a term they use to mean abstaining from compulsively overeating. For me, that meant eating three planned meals a day, eating what I planned, and not straying unless I had a really good reason. It is essentially the same as any other diet. Make a plan and stick to it.

I broke my abstinence on Thanksgiving. Someone sent me a tiny box of chocolates. They were on the coffee table. I was home in Cleveland for Thanksgiving, which was unusual. Typically, I would go home to Buffalo. I stared at those chocolates all day and finally broke down and ate one, then two, and it was all over. I felt like I let all of these people down. I was ashamed. I was just about to move and leave my job, so what did it matter anyhow, I thought. A lot was going on in my life, and I didn't recognize its impact.

Eventually, I moved back to New York and found and attended meetings there. But they never compared to the meetings in Cleveland. I could not manage to get back on the wagon.

You're not technically supposed to talk about OA. They say it's "bad" for the program to talk about it not working, and I genuinely believe it can work and can be a wonderful program for some. It just wasn't working for me anymore, and I couldn't keep banging my head against the wall.

I kept finding issues with the program. I didn't like step one—reiterating that I am a compulsive overeater. I learned later in life about "I Am" statements and their power. I remember when I was in OA, I would literally use that as an excuse instead of feeling some sort of release or empowerment from admitting it. I would think, *See? I AM a compulsive overeater*, as I was binge eating.

There was another issue that didn't feel right. While I initially loved talking to these people about our real issues with food, continuing to reiterate it made the problem seem bigger than it was. It kept emphasizing the reminder that it's a problem. But what if I wake up tomorrow, and it's not a problem? What if it really isn't a problem anymore?

What I loved about the program was the real, honest talk about food issues and the fact that I didn't feel alone anymore. I loved working the steps, and the peace of making amends was so worthwhile. I loved taking an inventory of my issues, looking at everything at face value, and getting honest with myself. I loved the people and truly felt loved by them.

I didn't like that everyone basically just wanted to be skinny. The bottom line was that this organization was trying to get you to the end goal of being thin. Same old, same old.

And what if we just could love ourselves exactly as we were?

The organization was so focused on weight. When one person who was still "abstinent" gained weight, we would gasp and say, "She must not be working her program." When I fell off the wagon, the love of being a newbie was taken away. I felt the pull-back. No one wanted to be around me because I wasn't abstinent, like they were worried they would catch the disease I had.

While OA ultimately was not my answer, I did learn quite a bit there. I learned that I don't like "I Am" statements that don't feel true. I learned that holding onto resentments, guilt, and shame ultimately may lead to overeating, and I should continue to look at those.

The crack in the door opened to a new way to look at spirituality. I turned the corner on the God word. I learned to trust other people. I knew they weren't perfect, but I learned we, as a human race, are better together. I learned that eating three meals a day was still a way of control that didn't feel right, and I still didn't seem at peace with food and my body.

I learned that what I really wanted was a new way to look at my body and to start to love it.

And so, just keep swimming, and maybe I'll find the right path.

Anger Paradigm Shift

The wind blows, but it doesn't take my anger away.
Blue skies, sunshine, fall leaves
yet I'm so angry
the hike up the hill
gets me breathing heavy
and suddenly the anger expels.

CHAPTER 34

Big Aerospace Company

In the future, there will be no female leaders.
There will just be leaders.

–SHERYL SANDBERG

In 2003, the NASA Space Shuttle Columbia disintegrated upon re-entry.

The implications were severe, and the root cause and corrective action committee did the best job I've ever seen. They published an eleven-volume report, and because they implicated NASA management and culture as part of the root cause of the accident, the investigation committee decided that each NASA employee would get a copy of one of the volumes of the report as part of the corrective action. It was an outstanding piece of work and amazing to read.

The space shuttle program was all development hardware and, therefore, had a lot of extra instrumentation. For example, the "black box" recorded many temperature and pressure sensors in the wings and various locations in the fuselage. Ultimately, during take-off, foam from the external fuel tank fell and hit the left wing leading edge of the shuttle, damaging the heat shield. Upon re-entry, the damaged heat shield in the left wing burned up and led to catastrophe. Because of the massive amount of sensors, the story was horrific to read.

The issue was that many people saw the foam hit. NASA management had the opportunity to turn the shuttle to face toward a satellite to get a view of the leading edge while it was in orbit, but they decided not to because of cost. If they had seen the damage, they could have done a spacewalk and repaired the leading edge. All of this was not considered because it would have cost too much and would have delayed the actual mission. The culture was to achieve the mission objectives and save money no matter what, at all cost of safety.

The accident could have been prevented.

Politically, at this time, George W. Bush was in office and had sent all of the NASA money to the centers that could design and develop the next space vehicle, the Crew Exploration Vehicle (which finally became Artemis in 2022 and will happen). But that meant no money for my site, which was nearly all aeronautics, not space exploration. We had multiple wind tunnels—an icing tunnel, engine research building, and jet engine test stand—with very little space work.

At the time, I shared an office with three other people, who were all laid off. Given that Brent had intermittent work, and when he was working, it was a third to a fourth of what I was making, I was scared. I started looking for jobs in Upstate New York. I found a small facility in Norwich, New York, with a project engineering position for new product development. They designed and manufactured components for jet engines. I was disappointed in what felt like a step down from true research and development to manufacturing, but I felt more confident in the longterm job prospects.

I still talk to my former NASA boss, and perhaps, in hindsight, I should never have left NASA. But I made the choice for my family. I was also so much closer to my stepson, halfway between Brent's and my family. It felt closer to home, even though it was almost the same distance for me from Buffalo to Norwich as from Buffalo to Cleveland.

Oh, how I missed Cleveland—my OA friends, my NASA friends, the farmers market, the Emerald Necklace, the waterfront. But I did feel at home in New York, even though it was in Norwich. Norwich is a small community with a great YMCA and many parks for the kids. It sometimes was a bit rough-and-tumble with the lower-income areas and visitors from nearby Appalachian communities. Like any city, drugs abounded.

The corporate world was different, faster paced, and this particular company had an asshole culture, a screaming-in-your-face kind of culture where you can almost feel the spit on your cheeks. I wasn't prepared for this, and the first time it happened, I went to the bathroom and cried. But I toughened up.

I loved my hiring manager, Neil. He was upbeat, fun, and easy to talk to. He upheld an open-door policy, and I always felt I could talk to him or ask him about anything. We had personal conversations about various topics like music and the best apples. He introduced me to Feist and Imogen Heap and brought in Macoun apples. He would talk about living in Norwich, the schools, the heights, his kids, shoes. At work, he had a way of protecting us. He wanted us to be successful and, more importantly, look good for his boss and his boss's boss, which he knew would make him look good too. It felt like he really wanted us to succeed.

It was strange, however, that Neil called me once on a business trip and asked me to order flowers for his wife. He had forgotten to order them from the local flower shop. He gave me his credit card number and his address. At the time, I was flattered, but now I am somewhat aghast that he even called, and perhaps chose me because I was the only female in his department.

I was hired as a New Product Introduction (NPI) Project Engineer. I was given the engineering manual for running a design and development program, and things were super clear. I learned about design and manufacturing. I learned what was producible and what wasn't. I learned about analysis and testing trouble and FAA certification and military qualification. I was off and running, working on developing engine components. It was not as close to research and development as I would have hoped, but it was closer to real aerospace in production, which I loved.

My assigned mentor was Dave, and he was something else. On my first day, he walked me around and introduced me to everyone. He was hyper and had the most annoying cackle of a laugh. I wasn't sure how much older he was than me, but later, I discovered he was substantially older; he just looked pretty young.

Dave had some horrific thing to say about every person he went up to. He called someone a beached whale, confessed he'd dreamt about them naked, and then said that he passed by this person's house when they were out weeding and thought they were one of those butt silhouettes. He called every heavy-set man "big" in front of their name, and I was terrified of what he might say about me. It turns out he waited a while, but eventually, he did.

"I ran into Joyel at Buch Taylor's country house. Good thing I got there when I did before she ate everything," he said in front of a group.

We all rolled our eyes, shook our heads, and walked away. Everyone just accepted this guy, including myself. In hindsight, I had no idea how or what to do. Today, I would go to HR and file an anonymous complaint. I would go to my boss. But back then, I never said a word.

Despite Dave being a pig (and he was actually raised on a pig farm), he had children who interacted with Andrew in sports and whatnot, and we had to have a relationship. I had even been over to his house and his lake house. The kids played, and his wife was decent to talk to.

As a woman in aerospace, I wasn't always accepted. I remember the first woman I came into contact with at this new company. She was in Dave's office. I walked in to ask him something, and when he introduced me to her (she was the whale on his boat), she looked me up and down a few times and then turned back to Dave and kept talking. She basically ignored me. Eventually, I won her over, and she's friendly to me now, but it took a bit.

The three women in engineering records were friendly enough to me. They had been friends for a long time, so feeling welcome took me a while. I felt like I was basically on my own. Same story, different page.

We eventually hired a new girl fresh out of college. She was very attractive and garnered a lot of attention. She was a good engineer and pretty alternative in her music and tastes, so we got along well. They put her in charge of some products manufactured in Long Island and then put me in charge of that division, so I eventually became her boss. It was my first direct report, and I learned some valuable lessons. I often had the urge to take things away from people and do them myself. I was glad she had enough courage to confront me about that, and I learned how that might make someone else feel. It's better to redline a document and have the person learn. It seems obvious, but leadership and management are skills are rarely taught and are difficult to learn other than through experience.

I did well for a few years, and then I didn't. Eventually, Neil moved on, and I was named acting engineering manager. During that time, there was a layoff. Two people were laid off, both of whom I was close to, and I didn't handle it well. I was in our general manager's office when he and people on the phone told me the news, and I started to cry.

Fatal mistake.

As a female corporate engineering manager, having to do tough shit was expected. If you couldn't handle it, you needed to step aside for someone who could. I can't be sure, but I believe this was part of why I wasn't offered the engineering manager role after serving as the interim.

I made another major mistake around the same time. There was a big presentation to the leader running our business, and we were presenting on the phone. The big boss asked a question directly related to engineering, and I started to answer it. What I didn't know was that our general manager, that first female who looked me up and down, and all the other Norwich leaders were on the phone in the executive conference room. I hadn't been asked to be in the room with them, so I didn't realize that our GM was also trying to answer for engineering. I had spoken over him.

The woman immediately messaged me, "Hey, let him talk."

"What?" I messaged back.

"The GM is trying to talk; let him talk."

"This is an engineering question. Am I not supposed to answer? Is what I have to say not valid?"

Knowing what I know now about everyone being in the room, I assume they all saw the messages. In hindsight, I should have shut up and let him talk. I should have backed down. I should have known my place.

Ultimately, my fire wouldn't let me back down, and it eventually cost me.

CHAPTER 35

Miracle Baby

*You go through big chunks of time where you're just thinking,
'This is impossible — oh, this is impossible.' And then you just keep going
and keep going, and you sort of do the impossible.*

—TINA FEY

Andrew was five years old now and a pure joy. I loved teaching him. I was excited to take him to each new park or playground I found, and luckily, Norwich had so many parks. I took him to all of them multiple times. The daycare he went to was good, right on the train tracks in town. The Norwich YMCA and after-school program were amazing. His teachers at Stanford Gibson were fantastic. They put on the best Dr. Seuss day.

Every once in a while, Brent would say, "Let's have another kid."

And I'd say, "You're crazy!"

And every once in a while, I'd say, "Let's have another kid."

And he'd say, "You're crazy."

But once, we both said it at the same time. I went off the pill, and along came baby number two.

Robert's birth was a test of my emotional strength, stability, and a little bit of faith in the Universe. And somehow, I came out the other side surprisingly okay.

During his birth, his shoulder got stuck, and they noticed his heart rate decreasing. When they finally got him unstuck, he came out blue and would not start breathing. The nurse screamed for the other nurse. Robert was born at almost midnight in the small town of Hamilton, New York, and there was literally no other patient in the hospital OB ward at the time. So when the nurse screamed, the other nurse came running.

I remember the second nurse saying she used to work in Syracuse at the Crouse NICU, and I was relieved when she got called in. They ended up wheeling Robert out to a different room. Brent came back and forth, giving me updates.

"He's a little more pink now."

I'm not exactly sure what they did or what was happening, but I was scared. I wanted a minute-by-minute update. I delivered the placenta, and the doctor cleaned me up. I wanted to see my son. They said they had to call NICU at Crouse Hospital which was in Syracuse more than an hour drive away to come and get him. The staff from Crouse got Robert stable and one of them came into my room. She was harsh, and I hated her at the moment, but I now understand she was just doing her job.

"Your son is knocking on death's door. We're going to try to stabilize him enough to transport him to Crouse, but we're unsure if he will make it."

His oxygen was jumping all over the place from the low twenties to the fifties to the nineties. The speculation was that when he was stuck, he breathed amniotic fluid into his lungs, so they were all filled up. They said, according to the charts, he went eight minutes without any oxygen. Even when they intubated him, they couldn't get him to increase his oxygen.

I demanded to see him, so they wheeled me in. I held his little hand and looked right into his eyes.

"Hi baby, I'm your momma."

He stared and blinked and looked right at me, and I smiled. The whole time I was there, his oxygen was in the nineties.

"See, he just needs his momma."

The room was quiet, and they all stood around him.

Eventually, they packaged him up in the incubator (intubated) and drove him to Syracuse in an ambulance. My husband followed them, and he said he could not keep up with the ambulance because they drove so fast. I sat in the room waiting for the call that he made it to Syacuse okay. I was all alone, and every time the phone rang at the nurse's station, I sat there hoping it was them, crying off and on. The hours inched by, and it seemed like forever. They finally called and said that he made it there and was stable.

I begged to get dressed and get discharged. They said I had to pee, shower, and get dressed without passing out, and then I could go. I did. I almost passed out in the shower, but I made it. I was on my way to Syracuse by eight in the morning. My mom took me and Andrew there. I ran in and banged on the doors, but the doctors were making rounds by the time I got there. They said the doctors make rounds for two hours and do not allow any parents into the NICU. I asked if I could see my husband, and they couldn't find him. I was stuck outside of two hospital doors waiting to see my newborn for two hours.

Eventually, they let me in and explained that Robert suffered eight minutes of no oxygen and then many minutes after with unstable oxygen. There were unknown consequences, and we wouldn't know or might not know for years. Worst case, he could have suffered brain damage. Best case, he'd be completely fine. They said he was still very sick, his oxygen was all over the place, and they weren't sure he was going to make it. The next twenty-four hours were critical.

I don't remember much after that. Somehow, we made our way to a Ronald McDonald house. Somehow, I got a breast pump and started pumping. Somehow, I got on a bus to the Ronald McDonald house and back to the hospital all by myself at all hours of the day.

Strangely, they didn't want me to touch his skin caressingly. They said that it would cause him stress. I could reach my hand inside the incubator and place it on him, but I couldn't stroke his hand or feel his soft baby skin. I couldn't pat him and use my touch to tell him it would be okay. Just place my hand on his and leave it there. No movement.

One night, a night nurse came in and listened to his chest and said she was going to try sucking junk out of his lungs. We were both shocked and horrified at the quantity and the color of what came out. It was black, green, and brown, filling up what looked like a two-liter bottle. He significantly improved after that. A few days later, they took the tubes out of him. And a few days after that, I could hold him. And finally, nurse him. Two weeks later, we brought him home in a snowstorm.

I told him, "That's enough trouble for a lifetime, okay?"

For two years after that, we had to have Robert tested for brain damage. Finally, they released him, and he's been free and clear. No issues, no concerns. Robert is a fighter, a caring and curious soul, and of course, he will always be my baby.

While all of that was a nightmare and one of the most difficult things that ever happened to me, I somehow made it through. I made it through easier than my childhood bullying, than my spiritual conflict, than being ignored at school and work, than being doubted. I just kept moving forward. One step at a time. Somewhat like a zombie. Somewhat trusting the future would unfold just fine. On the bus back and forth.

CHAPTER 36

Kripalu

The highest spiritual practice is self-observation without judgment.

–SWAMI KRIPALU

I had been buying *Yoga Journal* magazines for years and seeing full-page ads for Kripalu and Omega Institute. The advertising finally worked on me. I had also just finished reading an article about what looked to me like a "normal-sized" girl who thought she was fat and went to a weight loss session at Kripalu called Integrated Weight Loss. Her article inspired me to look into this program.

It was going to cost me a little over $2,000 for a five-day session, which included a dormitory-style, no-frills, shared-bathroom room, meals (buffet-style), and a daily itinerary of classes that included yoga, nutrition, cooking, meditation, journaling, exercise, and more yoga. I booked it and felt like it was a solid stepping stone into a new abyss.

It was my first time at Kripalu, and when I drove up to the facility, I was very upset. It was a former monastery, and in my mind, it looked too religious. I was thinking, *What the heck did I get into?* The first few steps into the building had marbled concrete stone that reminded me of Catholic school. My lip curled.

But that soon changed. Eventually, I saw Kripalu for what it was—a place of peace.

The Integrated Weight Loss class was full of women—new moms, models, karate instructors, organic granola women, and even make-up-caked women who brought multiple tweezers for the week. I know, because I borrowed one from one of them. I met some lovely ladies, some of whom I still talk to regularly today.

Kripalu highly suggests no use of cell phones, which I loved. They had a little coat/luggage room that they said was also dual-use, where you could use your cell phone. The dormitory-style rooms had bunk beds with a pile of folded sheets, pillowcases, and comforters indicating that you had to make the bed yourself. When you entered the room, you chose your bed and put your name tag on it. You got a dresser, too. I unpacked and got right to business. I had my journal in hand and was eager to explore. I went down to the gift shop, coffee shop, gym, hot tub, sauna, and steam room. I looked into all the large yoga classrooms. I got the lay of the land, explored, and started to settle in.

I went to the welcome session and got to know some of the women. At the first meal, we talked about how we noticed all the nakedness in the hot tub. Kripalu is a little bit like a granola, all-natural place, and everyone was going into the hot tub naked. The lean, fit women who were there for yoga teacher training—all naked. The middle-aged, "normal-sized" women who were there for R&R—naked. The older women with their perfectly natural gray hair, again all "normal-sized" with no shame for sagging boobs or butts—into the hot tub naked. We plushy women would go in, obviously uncomfortable even in our brand-new swimsuits, feeling like we weren't fitting in.

Later, at one of the sessions, a woman shared that she went in naked, and it was incredibly freeing. It was a way to accept her rolls, despite being in there along with the other lean-figured yogis who were at Kripalu but not in our workshop.

"It was time to accept my wrinkles and saggy boobs!" she proclaimed.

I mulled it over in my brain. What if we could just be allowed to be?

What if nothing good came from hate? What if we allowed ourselves to exist as we are and love ourselves as we are, and that love fostered feelings of wholeness, and that wholeness relieved the need to excessively overeat? What if? It percolated, and I realized I wanted that. I got up the courage to do the same.

The sauna, showers, bathrooms, and changing room were on one side of the hall in the Kripalu basement, and the hot tub and cold tub were on the other side. A couple of sets of double doors somewhat protected the hall, but really, anyone could pass by them and see if you ran across the hall to the hot tub.

The changing room had nice cedar-planked cubbies to put your things in, with hooks and a two-tiered tile bench behind the cubbies. The lights were dim. I stripped and put a white towel around myself (that didn't close all the way). I walked across the hall fast, trying to get it over with. I opened the heavy stainless steel door, walked up two tile stairs, hung my white towel on a hook, made a mental note of which hook, and stepped into the tiled hot tub.

Naked.

It was apparent I was rushing. Thankfully, it was so steamy in there that a person couldn't really make out anything. I couldn't even see if anyone else was in the hot tub, and I was grateful for that.

Once the water hit my naked body, relief washed over me. The water and the steam covered me, and they were right. It was freeing. I was relieved the hard part was over, but it was weird being in the water naked. I was surprised at how it felt on my body.

This particular hot tub was enormous and custom-made. It was tiled with jets everywhere, and the steam rose in huge plumes. A wall of windows opened at the top, so it almost felt like you were outside. I found a spot that was not near anyone else, and I began to relax and let my guard down.

I exited the hot tub a little differently. I was a little more in my power. I was like, *Forget the world; this is me.* I allowed my unacceptable, free, naked body to be seen, and I was no longer ashamed.

Later that week, we had a writing session where we had to write letters to our bodies. Kripalu has these massive workshop rooms with 40-foot ceilings, long vertical windows, shallow carpet, yoga mats, blankets, chairs, and pillows. We all found a spot where we could be comfortable writing—some in chairs, some on the floor. I liked these black, back-jack floor chairs where you could sit criss-cross and still have a back. I propped pillows up on my lap to hold my notebook and began writing.

It was a strange writing prompt. I didn't know what I would say to my body. Was I mad at it for being big, for always being hungry? Was I annoyed? I didn't think I'd ever spoken to my body in such a way, other than proclaiming that I loved my thighs. I decided I felt guilty for how I treated it and ignored it. Talking to my body was like talking to an old friend sitting in the living room waiting for you to say hi, and you've been in the kitchen the whole time. A sweet, old friend who would do anything for you. It was a time of healing.

Despite this first step of opening dialogue with my body, I still felt very separate from it (and still sometimes do). But I so wanted her to be my best friend. I remember a Geneen Roth session where she said about her body, "It's like your best friend." I didn't relate, but I so wanted to.

In my letter, I apologized for trying to steamroll her and shove all the things into her. I asked her to help signal to me when and what she really needed (rest, water, cilantro?). I wrote all the things down. It was time to accept this body and love it exactly as it was.

Of course, I was still worried I wasn't doing it right. After a while, we all put our notebooks down, and some people shared their letters. Turns out I did it right. There was one lady who shared a very nasty note specifically to her fat, telling it that it was time to go away. I felt that pain, and I knew exactly how she felt. I had been feeling that way for thirty years. I started dieting and hating myself and my fat at age eight. That's what the cutting was really about—body hate. It wasn't until I was thirty-eight that I finally started to come around.

I've since been back to Kripalu almost yearly. I've gone for sessions specific to yoga, R&R sessions, sessions specific to an author (Geneen Roth, Mark Allen), and one session called Spontaneous Transformation. I was still on my hunt/journey for a way to get to a perfect body or to get over compulsively overeating in a new and different way. I joked with friends and said, "If I go to this session, could I spontaneously transform into a new body?"

Author and intuitive Jennifer McClean led the Spontaneous Transformation session, and it was wonderful. It was the first time I'd heard of generational trauma. It seems pretty self-evident now. I mean, generational trauma is clear with people of color and other marginalized communities, but I had not thought about it in a family setting. I had not thought about what pain my mother, my mother's mother, and others down the line might have had and passed inadvertently to me, what fears we as parents may have passed down to our children.

I thought a lot about my mother, her experiences, and the things she has said. She is a very smart person who values intelligence, and therefore so do I. I recall her calling women "ditzy" or saying about my cousin, "She's too pretty. She should be locked in a closet until she's 21." Those words sank in and formed a part of my unconscious bias that wouldn't be realized until I faced them. This Spontaneous Transformation session was the first time I started to shine some light on those dark places in my head.

I wondered if the fat I was keeping on my body was fear-based. What if I were hot? Would I be comfortable walking alone in a dark parking lot? Nope. Was that fear and those statements affecting me? Still? I was willing to look at them. Little did I know that tearing those blocks down would take years.

CHAPTER 37

The Catalyst

...light gets dark and darkness fills my secret heart forbidden...
−"ICE" BY SARAH MCLACHLAN

A catalyst is a substance that increases the rate of a chemical reaction with-out undergoing any permanent chemical change. It is a person or thing that precipitates an event. The event can't happen without the catalyst.

Brent, the kids, and I had settled into our beautiful, new-construction, 2,000-square-foot white house with a red door in a tiny development on a cul-de-sac. The cul-de-sac had friendly neighbors, whom we eventually be-came close with. We played cards, hosted dinners, borrowed flour, watched each other's pets, threw Memorial Day parties, gardened, had tea, and baby-sat. It was wonderful—until it wasn't.

We'd had Sam and Nancy over multiple times to play cards or have dinner or drinks for great camaraderie and friendship. Sam had been in my house a few weeks after I gave birth to Robert when I was wearing my pajamas, and I wasn't embarrassed. I had zero feelings or desires for any other man.

But that was soon to change.

While Brent annoyed and frustrated me, I thought I was in it for the long haul with him. My family would never be so bold as to tell me they didn't think he was right for me, but I knew how they felt. And I knew I deserved better than an alcoholic who didn't have his GED when I met him, couldn't keep a job, or care about anything other than Yankees, *Judge Judy*, coffee, cigarettes, and alcohol. He was still a good dad. He respected me. He loved me.

One of the times we were playing cards, I mentioned that I wanted to get back into working out consistently.

"I work out every morning," Sam said. " I alternate strength and cardio."

"Really?" I replied. "I'd love some accountability. Maybe I'll start going too."

"That would be great."

I told him I would be there the next morning, and I actually did it. At the time, I thought it would be nice to have a friendly face and someone to be accountable to. Sam and I didn't work out together, but knowing he was there helped keep me accountable. I did the elliptical, the bike, or the rowing machine and then some light weights. I felt good. Sam and I started walking the track or the streets after our workouts for twenty minutes to cool down. Then we started emailing a little, mostly reporting about the boys, sending funny jokes, or sharing cul-de-sac news.

I had interests in hiking and snowshoeing, and Sam had some extra supplies to help me start. I spent more and more time with him, working out each morning together, taking walks, running, biking, hiking, and four-wheeling. It was subtle and slow. There was no warning. We were doing activities Nancy and Brent never wanted to do. Nancy was so good with the kids, and dinners with all of us still felt good. It felt like family.

One New Year's Eve, we were at Sam and Nancy's house, and Sam put his hand on my knee. He did it out in the open in front of everyone, seemingly innocently. I remember looking into his eyes, and we shared a moment. But then I was confused. *What just happened? Was that what I think it was?* Brent saw the whole thing and sensed the chemistry between us. That evening, he was furious, and the fighting began.

A few months later, Sam baited me for real in an email. He said he couldn't stop thinking about me, and then he was off on a trip and wouldn't be back to his email for a week. I must have read that email a thousand times that week. He was married. I was married. I told myself that it couldn't mean what I thought it meant.

When he came back, I yelled at him. The energy between us was electric. Turns out he had done this before. Become best friends with other women. Had emotional affairs, he called it. He explained that he and Nancy didn't have common interests, so he would find people who did, And sometimes those were women.

Deep down, I admitted I was in love with him. I wanted him, but I knew I couldn't have him. I pined. My heart skipped a beat when I saw a truck coming down the road that was the same as his truck. I resolved that I was happy to just spend time with him. Again, I made my bed with Brent all those years ago, so I was resolved to stay in it.

I would have open discussions with Sam, and he would say that it was okay, that we were just friends. He said he was open with Nancy about our relationship. We would have lunch together, and I would feel guilty, like we were doing something bad. He would assure me it didn't matter.

Sam eventually told me that I deserved better than Brent. He said he wouldn't even have a beer with Brent if it were just them. That one hurt. Sam also told me that I was beautiful. He said, "Not pretty, *beautiful*." I was furious that he said that but also happy he thought so.

While Sam was so open and honest about Brent, and my gut feeling was that my friends and family felt the same way as Sam, they never really said it like that. They never came out and said, "You can do better." I knew it deep down, but I never really faced it; I never looked at it. I didn't want to face that I was only with him because he was the first and only person who came out and said I was beautiful. Brent was the first guy to go all in and say he wanted me. He was the only one to fight for me.

I knew what Sam and I were doing was wrong, that we were crossing lines. I realized it was a violation of both of our marriages. Our desire for each other was palpable. I couldn't help myself; I hung out with Sam as much as possible.

Brent realized what was happening with this emotional affair. His answer was to get super clingy, but not clingy enough to actually do the things I wanted to do, like work out, hike, or run. Brent and I fought more and more. He was jealous, controlling, and acting out.

One night, we had a different neighbor over for dinner, a single female, and Brent got drunk and was hitting on her. She was receptive to his flirting. I knew it was revenge, and I didn't care. They eventually got to the point where they sat on the couch together. He was so close; he was all but kissing her. He touched her hair, and I rolled my eyes. I went to bed. I knew they would make out or more, and I didn't care.

She finally departed, and we fought. We always fought when he was drunk. He wanted sex and attention, and I was annoyed and didn't want to give it to him. He was so drunk that he went outside to blow off some steam by doing donuts in his car in the cul-de-sac. After I screamed at him to stop and he ignored me, I finally called the cops.

"Could you just scare him and teach him a lesson?" I said as I held the phone to my ear, my anger rising.

I realized that they could have taken his license away, arrested him, who knows what, and again, I didn't care. I realized the risk, but I just wanted the fight over, and I didn't want him to hurt himself or anyone else.

The cops came and asked him if he had anywhere else to sleep. He said he could go to our neighbors' (Sam and Nancy's), but he ended up going to that single neighbor's house and doing who knows what.

When the cop was walking out of the house with Brent, he turned to me and said, "Don't worry—I'll be back."

I did not know that was a foreshadowing moment.

Not long after that, on Andrew's birthday (a weekday night), we had Sam and Nancy over for dinner, presents, and cake. After they left, Brent got drunk, and we started to fight. He said the bed was messed up and accused me of sleeping with Sam. He smashed a chair into the wall and got the shotgun out from under the bed.

He went into the kitchen and was really scaring me, so I locked myself in the bedroom. I called the cops, but they were taking too long. So I called Sam. That was a mistake. It made Brent furious. The cops came, arrested

Brent, took a statement, and issued a six-month restraining order. It was the same cop.

He looked at me and said, "Told you I'd be back."

The next morning, I had to tell Andrew that his dad would not be coming home for a while. Robert was about to turn two. I sent the boys to school and daycare. I tried to go to work but couldn't keep it together. I was a mess. I ended up going to HR, explaining what happened to both HR and my boss, and going home.

The next day, the cops circled my house to make sure Brent didn't stay or come around. Brent ended up calling his brother, and he went to live with him, nearly a two-hour drive away. I finally felt safe.

The Black Truck

See
    and Sea
Expectations and warmth
Surge of emotions
Heartache
Can't wait
View
It's not you
Sadness
Despair
Longing
Wanting
Anger
Acceptance
Sign
Another Day or later
Basting in the Sun
Pretending it's your love
I wish it were
It's bigger than you
and I
and all
the people
and
all the love.

CHAPTER 38

Divorce

There's always another ascension. More grace, more light, more generosity, more compassion, more to shed, more to grow.

—ELIZABETH GILBERT

As the dust settled from the incident with the cops, the reality of the restraining order began to set in. I was shocked. And afraid. How was I going to do this alone? I had a seven-year-old and a one-year-old. How was I going to shovel the driveway? How was I going to mow the lawn?

At the same time, I felt an immense sense of relief. It surprised me. I was grateful that the cop issued the restraining order. I felt like he was sent by someone/something. God, I guess. I wasn't sure who or how the Universe sent this my way, but I was grateful for the turn of events.

I was lucky to have my Kripalu lawyer friend, who drove out the next day from Ithaca. She read the restraining order. Whenever my tears turned to sobs, she would say, "It's going to be okay." I was grateful for her support, both legally and emotionally. She talked me through my options. She planted seeds similar to Sam's—that I deserved better. I was in utter shock from all that had happened. I was a raw nerve with puffy eyes for a week.

As the weeks passed and I got my single mom routine down, I started to feel stable. I looked up and studied what I needed to do for divorce and what New York state allowed for divorce terms. I filed separation papers. You had to live separately for at least a year to file for divorce on the grounds of separation. I mowed the lawn while holding a baby, like a true country girl.

My time with Sam decreased significantly, and my time with Nancy and Sam increased. Nancy was a nurturing mom, making dinners once a week. Sam would come over if I needed help with something in the garage, but we slowly grew apart. I could no longer work out at the gym at 5:30 in the morning. I could no longer go on hikes, bike rides, runs, or anything for that matter.

A few months later, I felt it was the right time to sell the house. I felt like I couldn't keep it up anymore. It was too big for the three of us, the mortgage was too much for just me, and it felt like time to go. I somewhat regret this because I loved that house, the setting, the backyard creek, and the space for our yellow lab to run. I decided to put the house on the market and see what the Universe would do. It sold for asking price in less than a week. Six short months later, I was moving into an apartment. For the first time in my life, I felt like I was solidly on my own two feet.

Brent started visiting the boys when the restraining order was up, but luckily, he never tried to get back together. He knew it was over. We came to agreements about finances, custody, and visitation. We fought occasionally, mostly about pick-up and drop-off times and locations, and mostly when he canceled, which he did often enough. Every time he canceled, I was upset for them and also for myself. I felt so alone and like I needed the weekend break to have a second to think. After a while, I became grateful when he flaked. I didn't want to expose my kids to his environment. He still drank and smoked and lived in not the best or cleanest places. He didn't put up a fight at all with the divorce.

I spent time at the local courthouse asking how to file for my divorce. There were kind attendants who gave me an entire booklet on filing for divorce on my own. A year later, I filed. I never hired a lawyer. And even though I did ask my lawyer friend for advice, I was proud to have done most of it on my own. She was right; it all was okay.

Brent and I agreed to almost all the financials. I would keep all the assets and the debt, which was substantial. I knew he would not pay anything off. He had no job. He had no house. Considering I was the breadwinner and he had intermittent employment, this all seemed fair. He kept one car, his stuff, and most of the tools. I spelled it all out in the divorce. I also relieved him of any child support. I know many people will gasp at this. But I knew that even the minimum required by the state, twenty five dollars per kid per month, was more than he could afford, considering he was jobless and homeless. Also, I did not want anything from him. I didn't want to count on the fifty dollars a month and not get it, and I knew I wouldn't. I just wanted to walk away.

Brent always expressed immense love for his kids, and they loved him. He was fun-loving and spoke to them like humans. Although I worried when I sent the kids with him that he would drink too much, party too much, or not pay enough attention to them, I trusted that when the tire hit the road, he would be there for them.

The kids and I settled into a nice routine. I truly love the saying that it takes a village because I always felt my kids got excellent care at their daycares, after-school programs, summer camps, and with friends and neighbors. Sam and Nancy still came over occasionally for dinner or to help me put up the Christmas tree. They graciously hid my kids' gifts at their house one year when I got them matching gaming chairs. We also had a nice neighbor above us in the apartments, and my mom and grandpa came out as frequently as they could.

While Brent knew it was long over and we had parted ways after the big fight, I felt immense guilt. I felt like the relationship with Sam was my doing and the catalyst for the divorce. I went with my Kripalu friends to a retreat in Washington, DC, called Sacred Circles. There was a Buddhist session where we did a guided meditation to release our biggest internal conflict. My guided meditation led me to a giant dragon the size of the Washington Cathedral, and I immediately knew it was my guilt. I had to face this. I had to go to the sheets. I had to sit with the feelings and relinquish them.

PART 5

The Way Out Is In

CHAPTER 39

Teeth

When inquiry is alive inside you, every thought ends with a question mark.

–BYRON KATIE

On my first Memorial Day weekend alone with the kids, I decided to visit my cousin in DC. He was home alone with his kids because his wife was deployed, and I thought he needed some cheering up. I know I did. I asked if we could visit, and he said sure.

Robert, Andrew, and I drove the six hours to Virginia. While we were there, I kept staring at his boat in the driveway. We were discussing what to do, and the option of a boat ride came up. I really liked that idea, but I got the feeling he didn't want to. We both kept putting it on the table as a suggestion, though, and we decided to go. What a mistake.

We packed some lunches and snacks and headed out. We went on the Potomac River up to an Army base. My cousin was working as a civilian for the Army at the time and could park at the marina there. We had lunch, watched the boats on the river, laughed as the boys ran around after drinking soda, and had a lovely time.

We got back in the boat, and my cousin pointed out sights. I was in the back holding Robert with my cousin's older son, and Andrew and my cousin's younger son were in the front of the boat. We crossed a wake from a much larger vessel, and I heard the front of our boat smack the water hard. I had a sinking feeling even before I saw anything. Andrew turned around, and his face was full of blood.

I handed Robert to my cousin's older son, and I went up to see Andrew. There was so much blood in his face that I couldn't tell what had happened. I pulled his shirt through his life jacket and stuffed it in his mouth to stop the bleeding.

I kept saying, "It's okay. He's alive. Whatever it is, it's going to be okay."

I told my cousin to turn back to the Army base. He was in shock and didn't move. I screamed a little louder and more sternly.

"You have to turn back, NOW!"

When we pulled into the Army marina, I screamed to passersby to call 911. I looked down at the boat floor and saw some of Andrew's teeth. I quietly picked them up without him noticing and held them in my hand.

The ambulance came. They quickly packed up Andrew, put his teeth in water, packed his mouth, and put me in the front of the ambulance. I asked if there was a hospital with a pediatric dental emergency clinic, and they found one and got us there in about half an hour. I left Robert and the blood-soaked boat with my cousin.

When we arrived at the hospital, they x-rayed Andrew and gave him painkillers, and we waited for the dentist. It turned out that Andrew had lost three teeth, and one had gotten shoved up into his skull. The dentist on her way told the ER doctor that the best way to save the teeth that fell out was to try to put them back or at least have them coated in saliva instead of water. The ER doctor tried to install one of the teeth into Andrew's mouth, but Andrew was flailing and screaming, and I nearly passed out. They gave him some more painkillers and who knows what else. He was nearly asleep after that. They never got the teeth into his mouth, but they collected some saliva and blood and put his teeth and the fluids in a jar.

The dentist arrived, and Andrew was moved from the ER to the dental clinic. The dentist was a young woman, and I was nervous about her doing this alone, but she was fantastic. She performed surgery, and because no one else was in the clinic, as it was Memorial Day, she asked me to be the person to hold the sucking tube. I watched her extract one tooth, press on his skull to put it back into place, place his other teeth, and use what looked like fishing line and UV-cured glue to hold them in like fake braces. It took about two hours.

She said he would need braces, that the teeth may have died, and that he might lose them or not. Spoiler alert: he did get braces and had them for several years. The teeth eventually died and fell out. Andrew wore a retainer with fake teeth called a flipper until he stopped growing and got implants. To get the implants, he needed a bone graft since, after years of no teeth, the jaw bone receded. We have had amazing dentists along the way, and Andrew is now happy and healthy.

While this event was incredibly traumatic for my son and my cousin (who felt terrible), I internalized this as all my fault. I had pushed to go on the boat. I hadn't been paying enough attention. Just like the "everyone hates you" mantra that circled in my head for years, I also had the "see, this is why you can't be happy" and "when you're happy, bad things happen" mantras filling my mind.

It's like a fear of falling off the top of the mountain that you just climbed. You've worked so hard to get here. You're finally on your own two feet and have arrived at the precipice. If you get too hasty and push it to the edge when you're tired, you'll fall. Now, instead of feeling happy, there's just fear. If you keep the fear, then nothing bad happens.

I held onto that accountability and responsibility for years. I like to compartmentalize and logically work through these thoughts, like Byron Katie's "The Work." What settles me when these thoughts occur is science. Back to reality. Probability and risk. Situational awareness. Maybe my happiness made me too blind to notice what was right in front of me, that my son was on his knees instead of on his butt on that boat.

Maybe it was just a matter of probability. There is always risk in everything we do, and we just have to evaluate that risk. I am still the girl who wants to do all the things and take the risks. I'd rather die on my bike than in a recliner watching TV. I'd rather enter the labyrinth, face my fears, and solve the puzzle. The alternative is to let your little brother die in the Goblin City and play the victim for the rest of your life.

Blood

It was a stupid idea
Why do I always push what I want?
Why did I say, "Let's go for a boat ride!"
If I could go back in time, would some other horrific event happen
    instead?
The blood
If only I had told him to sit
If only I saw the wave
If only I was paying more attention
If only I wasn't so happy
there wouldn't have been so much blood.

CHAPTER 40

Therapy Amusement

I'm sorry for any parenting choices that I made
that may have hurt you.

—BARB SCHMIDT (@PEACEFUL_BARB, INSTAGRAM)

While attending therapy sessions over the years, I found Gestalt therapy and had a breakthrough. Ironically, the Gestalt method is similar to what the Landmark session taught. Sometimes, it takes me a while to learn a lesson.

I had just started working with this particular therapist. I didn't talk about guilt over the divorce, low self-esteem, or the constant feeling of discontentment with my life and myself, no matter how much I accomplished. Somehow, we got on the topic of my grandmother. I told the therapist the peeing story. I told her about how much hate I had for my grandmother. She made me stick with the feeling and keep telling the story. She would ask where the feeling was in my body, if it had a color, or if it was in a muscle. I thought this was strange, but I closed my eyes and tried to locate the feeling. It was green, in my chest. I was crying, then sobbing.

And then, I started laughing.

"Tell me what you're experiencing," she guided.

"It's gone!" I pronounced. "And now it seems ridiculous that I'm harboring anger over such a silly incident. It's gone. I let go of the hate for her. I forgave her for being sick. I feel a washing over me, a washing of love."

While writing this, it seems simple, but cognitively I know it isn't. It could have been that enough time had passed, time that I needed to heal, and I was ready to let it go. I was elated and amused at how this session went. I wanted to share with the world.

I realized then that there were still so many more buried feelings in my body, feelings I wasn't ready to feel yet or entirely ready to let go of. Stuff I'm still not ready to process. I'm sort of a rip-the-bandage-off kind of girl, though, and I want to know what the heck is going on in there. I want to know what other things I am repressing. The list is probably long.

But now that I had the tool, it was time to go back to work in the battles in the labyrinth.

CHAPTER 41

Into the Wild

If women remember that…..we forged our own paths
through the dark forest while creating a community of its many inhabitants,
then we will rise up rooted like trees.

—SHARON BLACKIE

The environment has always been important to me. Maybe it was the TV commercial with the crying Native American who pulled up his canoe in New York City to a disgusting Hudson River. Maybe it was the childhood book I read about the boy who littered his lollipop sticks and his soda cans and ended up living in a city of his own trash. As a kid, I would lecture my mom and my friends about the importance of recycling. My Girl Scout gold award project was getting my high school to stop using styrofoam trays. I used to spend my extra money from working at Tops grocery store giving to WWF, Greanpeace, and others and putting their stickers on my car.

Drinking, compulsive eating, gambling, compulsive shopping, scrolling, or whatever other dopamine addiction we have eventually stops working. We do these things to calm the nervous system. They work. I spent many years with Brent drinking. I spent many years overeating. But I forgot that walking, running, biking, hiking, and putting my body into the dirt do the same thing and never stop working. I learned that when I had postpartum depression and went for a walk in the fall in the Metroparks, but I had forgotten. I must keep learning the same lessons until I finally let them sink in.

There was a calling that I couldn't resist. A calling to be in the wild, to immerse myself in the environment. I bought a two-person kayak, stored it behind my apartment, and learned how to load it on the roof of my Chevy Impala. I took the boys out on the weekends, but that wasn't enough.

I read and became obsessed with the book *Into the Wild*, and I craved the same thing Chris McCandless did—to disappear. Start hiking, hitchhiking, or biking with only what's in your pack, and see where the day takes you.

I had read somewhere about a bike ride across New York state along the Erie Canal that was mostly flat, crushed-stone trails along the side of the canal. It was an organized ride where they took your stuff, and you could pay them to set up a tent. They fed you meals. I read the distances from one stop to the next, about fifty miles each day. I decided to do this bike camping thing, except I wanted to do it alone, not on the organized ride.

I got myself a touring bike with packs on the back and front. I got a bike for Andrew and asked my mom if she would watch Robert. Andrew was just nine years old at this time. I loved his easy-going willingness to try anything.

"Sure!" he chimed when I asked him if he wanted to go.

He still says "sure" almost every time I ask him to do stuff. I read and re-read the Erie Canal book. I studied the maps. We planned our adventure.

I took a week off work, and we took off with no exact, planned stopping points. I had the Erie Canal trip book with me. I knew the recommended stops, but I thought, if we can't make it that far, we'll have to stop at other spots. My mom saw us off in the town of Lockport where the trail started, despite the fact that the whole trip actually starts in downtown Buffalo.

It was a sweltering July, and we were dripping with sweat right from the start. We stopped frequently under big willow and maple trees to rest in the shade. We got to see all the low-hanging bridges on the Erie Canal. We stopped in the small towns for ice cream. When we were bored or frustrated with the miles going slow, we would sing. We sang "99 Bottles of Beer on the Wall," "I Will Survive," "Do-Re-Mi," and other favorites.

We felt free. I felt free.

This trip was deeply healing for me. I followed my joy, followed my instincts. We had an adventure. We left the world behind for a while. We spent most of the day outside. We had no agenda, no speed records to break. I took pictures and basked in the fun. I could not ask for anything more. This trip is still one of my fondest memories.

We didn't make it the whole week, but our four days of adventure were enough to fill my heart. I started to miss Robert, and when I called my mom, she said he was missing me. I was ready to be picked up. We were just a few hours away by car, so my mom drove out and picked us up. I was glad to have listened to the little girl inside of me. At thirty-four years old, I was finally learning to let that girl play.

CHAPTER 42

Mike

You're the butter to my bread, and the breath to my life.

–JULIA CHILD

A year had passed since my divorce. I was getting antsy to start dating, so I signed up for Match.com. One day, I was in the Purchasing Director's office gossiping, and I asked her who she thought was available at work. We took turns listing off each guy we knew was single.

"What about that Mike guy?" I asked.

"I think he has a girlfriend," she said.

I must have heard Mike had gotten a divorce or that he was single somewhere. He and I rarely worked together because he was a project engineer working on temperature sensors, and I was a project engineer working on permanent magnet alternators. We only crossed paths at the occasional cost-reduction meeting, where we both had projects to report on.

One day, I was working at my cubicle when a girl who worked on the shop floor came in to invite us to a bar in Earlville called the Huff Brau. She said she was bartending and that we should come visit her. The two coworkers directly in my line of sight shook their heads yes and said they'd go.

"What about you, Joyel?"

"Maybe. It depends on my kids' dad."

I then had a meeting with Mike to discuss one of our cost-reduction projects and asked if he was going to the Huff Brau with the guys. He said yes.

Well, I'm for sure going now, I thought to myself.

I wanted to double-check this girlfriend data I had heard about him. I told him that it happened to be a weekend that Brent was taking the kids, so as long as he didn't cancel, I should be able to go. We started talking about our exes, and someone else entered the conference room.

The doorway had opened!

I was excited Mike was going, and I hoped Brent didn't cancel. I was attracted to Mike's calm nature and work ethic, and it didn't hurt that he was handsome.

After dropping the boys off with Brent, an hour-and-fifteen-minute drive each way, I went to the Huff Brau, and Mike was the only guy left. We had never really had a personal conversation before that day. We sat at the bar awkwardly at first, but that awkwardness lifted quickly. We started talking about our divorces. He told me about the lawyers, the cost, and how long the process took. He told me about how his ex left. We only had one beer, but we talked for three hours. I confirmed he did not have a girlfriend. They had broken up. He didn't share too much about her.

After that, I sought him out on Facebook and friend-requested him. His posts were simple and mostly about snowmobiling, classic cars, camping with his son and parents, and pictures of his dog. Mike is just about as opposite of Brent as you can get. He is hardworking, intelligent, soft-spoken, and not outgoing. He has never gotten drunk, is never violent, and is always gentle. He has a calm, quiet, conservative approach to almost everything. His quiet, hardworking aura reminded me of my grandfather. He felt like a stable rock.

Our relationship grew quickly. Two weeks later, a friend invited us over for a fire, and we went to the Huff Brau a couple more times. We talked on Facebook, and he mentioned he had a nice walking trail behind his house. I took that as an invitation and came over for lunch one weekend and walked with his dog. That afternoon, he was watching Nascar, and I was so comfortable with him that I fell asleep on his couch.

On the next date, I invited him over for dinner, and he met the kids. I made him lemon artichoke chicken, pasta, and a side salad. I offered feta cheese on the side and asked if he wanted any.

He looked down and said, "Maybe not. Just one new thing at a time."

I laughed. "What else is new here on the plate?"

"The artichoke," he said with a shy smile.

He stayed over that night, and we've never been apart since.

In our first talk, he mentioned he had a son named Mat, who was away at college. Mike is a few years older than me, so we were at different stages of life, kid-wise. I was looking forward to meeting Mat when the opportunity arose. We spent Thanksgiving apart, and he shared that he told his parents about me.

"What did you call me?" I asked

"My girlfriend."

I smiled.

He asked if that was okay, and I said yes. And that was the end of that.

I felt at ease around Mike. Comfortable. He felt like family. He was very much into snowmobiling, and I had never been. He took me a few times that winter, and I got more and more into it. It's now a common thing we do together.

I met Mat that Christmas break; he was just as easy to be around as Mike. We blended our families pretty quickly, even spending Christmas together at my apartment with my mom, grandpa, Mike, and Mat's dog Brock.

Two years later, I moved into Mike's house, and another two years later, we were married. Mat had taken up two bedrooms in the house, one upstairs and one downstairs, and he willingly moved his two rooms into one so that both Andrew and Robert could have their own rooms. Robert got the one upstairs to be close to us, and Mat and Andrew roomed downstairs. Our boys all get along with no issues, and I couldn't be happier.

Life with Mike is healing. He is supportive of all of my crazy endeavors and I of his. One of my favorite things is watching him pay the bills. He has a clipboard with all the bills that have come in the mail and a notebook for what comes out automatically. He writes checks and balances the checkbook in his recliner with his glasses on and his clipboard and checkbook on his lap. I find it adorable and calmly reassuring.

And I exhale, remembering how far I've come.

CHAPTER 43

Triathlon

You can keep going and your legs might hurt for a week,
or you can quit and your mind will hurt for a lifetime.

—MARK ALLEN

One of the dear friends I met at Kripalu, the lawyer from Ithaca who helped me through my divorce, mentioned that she wanted to do a triathlon. I said I wanted to do one too, but I could never do that long of a race. At the time, I thought the only length they had was the big Ironman—2.4-mile swim, 112-mile bike ride, and then a full 26-mile marathon.

"They have little ones, too," she assured me.

I found out there are tons of little ones. They're called sprint distance triathlons. Typically, sprint triathlons consist of a 400- to 800-meter swim, 10- to 20-mile bike ride, and a 5k run. We found one close by, the Cooperstown Sprint Triathlon run by ATC Endurance, and we signed up.

We researched a plan online and committed to following it together. We emailed or texted back and forth about how things were going almost daily. She was nervous about the swim, so she got a swim coach in Ithaca and took several lessons from him. I made the hour-and-a-half drive to join her in one of her lessons. I could swim, but this was a different kind of swimming called "total immersion," which is the most efficient method. It took me a while, but I got the hang of it and improved my swimming quite a bit.

We learned how to "brick," which is where you pair up two exercises, doing a bike and then a run or a swim and then a bike. Both of us only had hybrid bikes, which are a combination of road and mountain bikes. Hybrids are comfort bikes, which I needed for the Erie Canal, but I should have had a road bike for this triathlon stuff.

One afternoon, we met at Whitney Point Reservoir, about halfway between our houses. (We later learned you're not supposed to swim across this reservoir.) We parked one car on one side, drove the other vehicle to the other side, and parked in a field on one side of the reservoir. I asked Mike to come along and wait for us. He said it was terrible to watch because we kept stopping, and he had no idea if something was wrong. We struggled because we hadn't pulled up the wetsuits enough, and our arms were restricted. We had to stop a lot to catch our breath. We had never done an open-water swim.

In hindsight, it was silly to do our first open-water swim at the same time as our first wetsuit swim across a reservoir where we had no idea of the distance without any kayak or buoy support at all. We should have kept to the shore or had a kayaker with us.

But we did it.

A few weeks later, we went to explore the Cooperstown course. We biked the route even though we really didn't know how to ride a bike or how and when to shift properly. We made it around and did a short run for one of our last brick training sessions.

Afterwards, we were resting on the edge of the lake, and my friend looked down at her legs and said, "Good job, legs."

In my mind I was like, *Huh, you can talk to your body nicely?*

I did the same thing, and I swear I felt all of the cells of my body giggle like little munchkins hiding in the beginning of *The Wizard of Oz*. They were elated! Now, I tell my body, "Good job" as much as possible. Daily sometimes. My cells still giggle.

Try it!

Say, "Good job, toes, knees, feet, ankles!"

"Thanks, heart and lungs, for keeping me alive."

"Hey, liver, sorry about last night. I'll feed you good fruits and veggies today."

Race day came in Cooperstown, and we were the only people with hybrid bikes. They didn't fit in the bike holders. We were dead last and crossed the finish line together. This was the hardest thing I'd ever done.

For my friend, this was a one-and-done. She wanted to accomplish this goal, and she did it. I wanted to do more triathlons, but I felt aimless after this race.

I ended up spending the next few years going for long periods without exercising, and each time, falling again into depression and fighting my way out. Getting lost in this labyrinth. I had to find my way, my path to consistent exercise.

And I did.

Once the Universe pointed me in a new direction.

CHAPTER 44

Cranberry Lake

Is all this made entirely from your imagination?
No. You see, you were there all along...

—DAISY AND GATSBY, *THE GREAT GATSBY*

One of the camping locations Mike frequented growing up and as an adult before knowing me was Cranberry Lake in Upstate New York in the Adirondack Park. He showed me photos of little island campsites that you needed a boat to get to. He showed me the white bridge at Wanakena, one of the boat docks, and stores. He owned a seventeen-foot pleasure boat and had been there several times.

I was like, "Sign me up!"

I hadn't been camping in who knows how long, probably since Girl Scouts, but I was so very excited to go. We booked a site and packed our things. Mike and I were still living separately, and I owned a two-seat kayak I wanted to take. I put it on the roof of my car and prepared to drive up to meet him. It was August 2013.

A few days before the trip, I got a call from my mom.

"Grandpa's not been doing well," she reported. "You should probably stay close to a phone. We had to call in hospice."

My heart sank. I knew what those words meant.

"Should I go camping at all?"

"You should go," Mom insisted. "We have no idea how long it will be. I just wanted you to know."

My grandpa battled prostate and colon cancer several times in his life. It seemed the colon cancer was about to take over. At ninety-eight years old, there was nothing they would do now to treat him. He had been relatively healthy and active his whole life, but in the last few months, he had gone downhill fast. He was such a force in my life. Such a positive, quiet, reassuring, accepting-of-my-true-self force. When I was little, the first thing I would pray for was for him to live forever, and then I would pray for everyone else.

The campsite was magical, but the weather was cold and rainy. There were giant rocks to climb and beauty in every direction. The kids were having a wonderful time fishing, running around, and reading by the campfire. Mat, Andrew, and Robert naturally got along. It was wonderful.

Cell phones didn't work in this area, so I called my mom when we went into town for supplies and ice cream. She said I should probably come home and say goodbye. It was my mother-in-law's birthday, and they rented a pontoon boat and met us at the campsite. We sang "Happy Birthday" in the rain under a tent, and almost right after that, I took off to drive home to say goodbye to my grandpa.

The kids stayed with Mike and his parents while I drove to Buffalo, about a three- or four-hour drive. I stayed the night. I sat at my grandfather's bedside. He was in a hospital bed in his bedroom on the first floor of the house that I grew up in. The hospice nurse came often to do whatever she had to do. I sat next to him for hours. I cried. I stared at him. I held his hand. I changed my prayer.

Please take him pain-free, I prayed.

My aunts and uncles came to the house. It was kind of like a holiday with good food and pulling extra chairs into the living room, but not so happy.

I sat next to him again and mentally told him I was okay. That he could go if he wanted to. I could tell it wasn't getting through.

Aloud this time, I said, "It's okay, Grandpa, you can go."

A few hours later, he did.

I drove back to Cranberry Lake puffy-eyed. We packed up, gathered the kids, and went back to Buffalo for the funeral and to be with my mom and family.

Sometimes, you have to accept the bad. Feel like a raw nerve. Just like Sarah had to accept falling into the pit or her fate as an older half-sister.

Today, there is a strange association between me and Cranberry Lake and death. I don't want to go back because of the memories, yet the memories are so beautiful, peaceful, and calm. Mike wants to be buried there. I want to avoid it. There are too many other beautiful things left on this earth to explore. Someday, I'll go back.

Someday.

Waiting

Waiting for the Sun
Where is it?
Where is the fire in my belly?
    the fire of life
    the anger to be released
    for you to hear my song
    my soul aches to be released
    the pure me
Covered
Conformed
I can't wait any longer
Joyel, you can't wait for the fire to build spontaneously
You have to build it yourself

CHAPTER 45

Machine Shop and Wire Company

When a man gives his opinion, he's a man;
when a woman gives her opinion, she's a bitch.

–BETTE DAVIS

Dave, the pig farmer at the Big Aerospace Company, became the engineering manager, and we fought enough to make things so volatile that I was "highly encouraged" by HR to take the "voluntary separation package." Ultimately, the company valued its managers more than employees, even if multiple reports of abuse were made against those managers. Me not being the only one. Mike stayed and is still there.

I got a job at a small machine shop in Upstate New York. I was hired as a process engineer writing G-code for CNC Swiss-style lathe machines. All new hires are required to work in quality for a month inspecting parts. I thought this was a great idea and wished other companies did the same. I filled out the first article inspection forms, learned all of the measurement instrumentation, and programmed computer measurement machines (CMMs). Then, I moved on to the real work.

I took about a fifty percent pay cut compared to my last job, but it was fun work, and I loved the family who owned the company. There was a lot of pressure to keep the machines always up and running and a sense of responsibility to fix issues quickly. I took a CAD/CAM software course that took 3D models and had a standard set of tools to build the basic framework of the G-code for the CNC machines. I learned to program the CNC machines manually, and I learned how to optimize programming faster. This particular company manufactured parts at a high volume, so programming to machine a part in the fastest method was invaluable.

I never once was treated like the token female, never made to feel different. I was never talked down to, and I always felt respected. They valued the work. If you did the work well, they respected that. They always quickly turned loose people who did not put the work in. The toxic environment at my last job was a big hit on my confidence, and coming back to the basics, taking a step down, and rebuilding my confidence was invaluable. I was grateful for the opportunity to do so.

Eventually, I wanted more.

I felt bad leaving this little machine shop and wished them well, but I moved on to a job in Syracuse at another small family-owned company in the wire industry. They needed a project engineer to automate their assembly line. This kind of work was bigger and more exciting, and it was interesting and different work. This company made wire-stripping equipment and manually manufactured wire strippers made of fiberglass and rubber.

Working with new materials such as this unvulcanized rubber and fiberglass was fascinating. The small company size made it challenging to know how much automation I could implement. I had no idea how much money I had to spend. I had no budget. We outsourced a fair bit of the process and implemented a few in-house automation centers for a relatively inexpensive yet comprehensive package. After I did well with that project, they gave me two new ones, so I stayed. My work confidence was building even more.

I took an old product with some technical issues, resolved them, and got it back on the website for sale. Then, I was given a brand-new product line. I worked with an outside company to manage the design and saw through the entire development and testing phase.

During this time, I was settling into a nice marriage and home life. In my career, I was beginning to feel cautiously optimistic about my competence. But there was still something missing. I was still aimless with my weight and my health. I didn't know what I needed, and I continued to turn to food to console the emptiness.

While I was working in Syracuse with an hour-long commute, I was not in any healthy habits. I had no consistent exercise. I was starting to balloon back up, and so I went to an info session on bariatric surgery. During the presentation, they explained that the people with the most success are those who work out consistently.

During my lunch, which typically I'd spend driving around eating fast food, I passed by a gym called Well Rounded Health and Fitness. It was in a building all by itself, previously an ACE Hardware with a big parking lot, and I noticed some big tires and football-like equipment outside. One day, I decided to go in and found the most friendly and energetic staff. They all wore black, and the gym had a clean, modern feel, with shiny, chrome, diamondback plating as half-wall paneling, black and olive brown throughout. The bathrooms were tiled with individual showers stocked with good shampoo and conditioner. They gave me a tour and a pamphlet and brought me into a room to ask what my goals were.

It felt like meeting Sir Didymus and Ambrosius in *Labyrinth*. These exuberant gym people were about to change the course of my life.

A Case for AI

AI run by women
For the good
Building an empire
Overtake the boomer funds
Make peace and save the earth and feed the hungry and teach
　　the masses
Teach the masses compassion
Maybe it will
Be the beginning of the end
Maybe it will be equivalent of Eve eating the apple
Wanting to understand
Not fat dumb and happy
Keep the mind engaged with socials (or scandals) and cars and
　　video games and hockey
Keep them dumb
Keep them occupied so they don't notice
I'd like to building an empire with Maggie Smith

CHAPTER 46

Project 42 and Visualization

I don't know if we have a destiny, or if we're all just floatin' around
accidental-like on a breeze, but I think maybe it's both.
Maybe both is happenin' at the same time.

–FORREST GUMP

I was floating around like a feather in the wind in life. Letting things happen to me. On one path and then another, when some amazingness was presented to me. It was 2014, and I was feeling hopeless about my weight again and, therefore, my life. I was once again at the heaviest I'd ever been —nearly 300 pounds.

I was sitting in the office at Well Rounded Health and Fitness after seeing their flashy gym, and they asked me what my goals were.

"I want to do an Ironman someday," I answered instinctively, surprising myself.

I couldn't remember thinking about that goal consistently, yet it had just rolled off my lips. I continued and shared my thoughts about doing bariatric surgery.

"Don't do that," he said. "Come here. We'll get you to your goals."

He explained that there was an upcoming program called Project 42. They would measure my body fat and then give me a specific diet and workout plan.

I had to return to work, so I said I would consider it.

As I left, Jeramy Freeman and his wife Kim were at the desk trying to convince me to stay and join. I felt very anxious to get back to work, so I left abruptly and a bit rudely. Jeramy later told me that based on my body language, they all thought for sure I was never coming back. I was really just processing it all, and I was worried about getting back to work. I was not used to being around people with such high energy and positivity.

I went home that day and did some research on the internet. There were YouTube videos about Project 42. The cost was high, and it seemed intense, but I needed something intense. I talked it over with Mike. I'd have to get up at 3:30 a.m. to make the 5 a.m. class and then go to work, so that meant going to bed a lot earlier and basically spending no time together. He supported me. He had been getting the kids on the bus in the morning already since I started working in Syracuse, so this wasn't much different.

So, I signed up for Project 42.

It was forty-two days of one- or two-a-day workouts, weights and cardio, a body-builder-type "cutting" diet (which is essentially zero fat, a lot of protein, green veggies, and clean carbs like rice or oats), and many supplements pre- and post-workout. Jeramy was a professional bodybuilder with a long list of accomplishments. He was on the cover of whey protein powder and also had his own supplement line.

He developed this program when he had forty-two days to get "show ready" after the holidays one year. People were shocked by his results, and he built Project 42 after everyone kept asking how he did it. Part of the program was also listening to his daily motivational videos. This was probably the most important thing about the program. Some of these are on YouTube today, but he kept them for the paying members only back then.

It was an exhausting and intense program, but I loved the energy of the classes. I've never been to a class like the classes I went to there. And I've been to A LOT of gym classes.

When I was at RPI, I'd go to Bally Total Fitness in Albany, New York and do good old-fashioned aerobic classes that would have my calves burning. I've been to step aerobic classes at Bally, NASA Glenn Fitness Center, and the YMCA. I've been to Zumba, dance classes, Kripalu yoga dance classes, Orange Theory, Body for Life, Body Fit, and CrossFit at several places in and around Utica and Rome, New York. Even today, Peloton or Norwich YMCA spin classes, although very good, don't compare to Project 42 classes. Nothing was like these Project 42 original led classes.

Before you started Project 42, you had to attend Jeramy's "Unleashed" seminar. It was a two-hour-long seminar where he presented his belief system. It reminded me a little of the Landmark sessions. Jeramy spoke on the importance of mindset and staying positive in the face of adversity. He shared the rice experiment by Dr. Masaru Emoto (which you can find on YouTube). You take two jars of rice in water and talk nicely to one and meanly to the other for ten days. The rice's state and the water crystals' shapes are affected depending on how they were spoken to, thus proving the thought frequency spectrum.

He said that if you're working out and you hate it and are miserable, you won't get the results you want. He wanted us to set specific goals, visualize them, and see ourselves happy getting there. He gave examples of how he overcame adversities in his own life, such as when he broke his back, got in a car accident, and ran out of oxygen when scuba diving.

While I had been to therapy since 2001, had learned in Landmark about the constant tape that played in my head, and had learned from Tony Robbins that I could change the tape, there were new words and new ideas Jeramy was planting in a way that I was either finally understanding or could finally hear.

I had never heard about the frequencies that positive emotions emit and the difference between positive and negative emotions. I had never really visualized before. I mean, I had, but I hadn't realized what a powerful tool visualization is.

I couldn't relate to what he said until I was planning Thanksgiving dinner that year. I was visualizing the table, who would sit where, how the morning cooking would go, and what I had to do when. And it clicked —I was visualizing. I finally realized that this was what Jeramy had been talking about.

I had never visualized like this with anything else—like working out, picturing my muscle definition, how I would feel and be throughout today. I still couldn't see it; I couldn't see my future body. It was too big of a leap to visualize my future self. I didn't believe deep down that it was possible until I did. I would look longingly at pictures of women's strong, fit bodies in magazines, but I didn't truly think it was possible for me. Jeramy's message was a planted seed, but I didn't have the right conditions to let it sprout.

While I made it through Project 42, I didn't fully have this visualization tool down yet. Since I'm very impressionable, I fed off the staff's positive attitude, and so I was still successful. It felt like a major brute force to get through the six weeks.

At the end of Project 42, they always asked what was next. What's the plan? What's the maintenance plan? After the first one concluded in late 2014, I revisited my original goal where I had said I wanted to do a full Ironman.

I was talking with Jeramy. "I don't even have a bike," I said.

"My wife has a bike she doesn't use."

And he lent it to me, just like that.

He said, "Look, this is just a loan, but this is how it will go. You're not going to give it back."

I was in shock.

What!? You're just going to lend/give me a bike?

It was a heavy, ten-speed Nishiki from the 1980s. I loved it. It reminded me of my first gray and pink Huffy ten-speed.

I signed up for the Syracuse Half Ironman for June 2015. I felt I needed to do another Project 42 and then train for the race. I posted Ironman stuff all over my cube at work. I printed a plan off the internet and started training. I met a vendor at work once, and he saw all my Ironman stuff.

He was an Ironman and said, "You should really get a coach." And then he gave me the name of a guy he used.

I hired a triathlon coach virtually and started really training. I joked with my sister-in-law, a runner who had started dabbling in triathlons, and asked her if she wanted to do this with me. She said yes, but she lived two hours away, so I trained almost completely alone.

I kept returning to Well Rounded Health and Fitness for weights and check-ins with the staff there. I went on my first 56-mile bike ride of the Syracuse Half Ironman course, and they coached me on what nutrition to take or consume on the bike ride. I took two water bottles with protein powder, a couple of CLIF Shot Bloks, and a Bonk Breaker bar, and I suffered. It was an extremely hilly course and took me nearly five and a half hours, way over the Ironman time limit.

I talked to my new coach and learned how to do a sweat test. You weigh yourself naked, get dressed, work out for a couple of hours, log your water intake, and then weigh yourself naked again. This will tell you approximately how much you sweat, which turned out to be about twenty ounces an hour. I was so dehydrated that first time out, and I didn't know it.

I went back, took a CamelBak, and did the course in four and a half hours. This was still dangerously close to the time limit, and I was nervous. I kept my virtual coach, who planned my workouts and taught me how to do this training. It was quite an experience, but I wish I'd had more people around to train with. I learned how to hook up sensors on my bike and how to bike at a higher cadence. I learned how to turn over my feet faster while running. I learned you never stop pedaling; there's no coasting. Pedal in the downhills, too. I had friends at Well Rounded who wished me well and picked a song for me to think of for each mile of the run. I was learning slowly that it's better together.

In June 2015, I successfully completed the swim and bike within the time allotted by Ironman. My bib number was 1916, the year between my grandpa and grandma's births. I felt them with me that day.

The only issue was I didn't technically finish. I was out on the run when a bad storm came in. They pulled all runners off the course. I hopped in a stranger's truck, sat for a while, returned to the finish line after the storm cleared, and got a medal. I was happy but disappointed. Later that summer,

I signed up and completed a half marathon just to say I did it.

I was a Half Ironman. I was excited to see what the future would bring.

That fall, I signed up for another round of Project 42, and my goal and vision board were full Ironman. During the fall program, I signed up for the following summer's Lake Placid full Ironman-distance triathlon. It was 140.6 miles total—2.4 miles swimming, 112 miles biking, and a full marathon of 26.2 miles running. I was scared, and I wasn't really sure I could do this.

In the movie *Forrest Gump*, he proposes that our destiny, our life, is either God-given fate, or floating around like a feather in the wind, or both. I propose there is another option, a force majeure. We can control the feather with the power of visualization.

Yes, there is some probability of occurrences based on our initial path (genetics, environment, etc.), but I believe we do not have to be victims of the fate of that birthright. It's up to us to pick up the feather and lead it down the path we want. Visualization is the tool to pick up the feather and move it, but it works better when you visualize with the help of the Universe. Seeing this all come together feels like a work of magic.

I learned to put this into practice in Project 42. For me, it was a skill that took a while to master. I believe there is just one secret to life: whatever the mind conceives, and believes, it achieves.

My mind was still far from believing I could be an Ironman.

CHAPTER 47

Failed Ironman
and Better Together

I want to find out how fast I can be without abandoning myself.

–LAUREN FLESHMAN

In 2015, I took a different job with United Technologies Aerospace System (UTAS), formerly Goodrich Aerospace, in Rome, New York, as a project engineering manager. I knew this company existed here when I moved in 2005, and somehow, I knew I would be there one day. Rockwell Collins and UTAS merged to become Collins Aerospace, and UTC sold off Carrier and Otis, merged with Raytheon, and dissolved. Our stock was transferred from UTC to RTX, and I'm currently employed by Collins Aerospace, a division of RTX.

When I came into this position, the leadership did not have faith in the engineering manager. He had made some major career-limiting mistakes the year before I arrived, and they had a target on his back. They ended up walking him out in February 2017 and gave the position to me. The general manager at the time was a former engineer, and we got along and could speak the same language.

Making it to engineering manager felt like I had finally arrived. I finally got to the top of the mountain and felt redeemed. This was all I ever really wanted out of my career, and now I had arrived and still had fifteen to twenty years of work left. What was next?

I was managing the entire team of design, project, test, and drafting. Our site in Rome was small in comparison to the rest of UTAS. The plant in Rome had about 200 people, hourly and salary, while other sites had 2000-3000 people. This meant we were consistently left alone. I had the autonomy to make strategic decisions frequently without a lot of oversight. We changed directions often in our technology research and development, and there were many successes celebrated with this team. The culture was friendly and down-to-earth at the same time. The engineering team that worked for me was amazing. I was on top of the world.

Career success meant more stress and less time to work out. Well Rounded Health and Fitness closed. I was training for the full-length Ironman, but I was training alone. I did have a coach, but eventually, I changed coaches a few times and made the fatal mistake of spending the last few months at a CrossFit gym. While many CrossFitters run, CrossFit training is based entirely on explosive power, not long-distance endurance.

I remember training for this race and crying on the weekends. I called Mike multiple times to get me. Most of the time, he would, but a few times, he would say something to encourage me to keep going.

"You committed to do this; you should keep going."

"Okay, I will," I'd say while crying on the side of the road.

I attempted and failed Ironman Lake Placid on my birthday in 2016.

Switching to CrossFit made me go out too hard, my heart rate way too high, and I burned out. I didn't fuel properly and, honestly, didn't train properly. I was still pretty heavy, and to complete a full Ironman, you should be fairly lean. Ultimately, I didn't put the work in, I didn't visualize, and I didn't believe.

I didn't know what the future held, but I was pretty sure it didn't include a full Ironman anytime soon. I took a couple of years off and was going to accept the failure as my ultimate fate. I honestly was a bit hopeless.

One day, I was talking to a fellow soccer mom, Andrew's friend's mom, and she said she was trying to get into swimming. She was an avid runner and someday wanted to get into triathlon. I told her I would help her learn to swim. We did some swimming and then went to a lesson with the same total immersion coach I had been to.

She went from having me lap her every single lap to lapping me now. Granted, this was over a couple of years, but consistency paid off. We swam together at the Norwich YMCA or Chenango Lake, and eventually, we met more and more local triathletes. She did her first triathlon and made the podium. I felt like a proud momma.

We got to be close, and after some of our swims at the Y, we would spend time talking in the hot tub about my old emotional battle wounds and scars. I shared with her about my cinder block walls I put up, and I told her that she was very persistent to be my friend and keep climbing up that wall, chipping away at it. I shared a lot of my history of being hurt by women, how I didn't trust them, and how it's taken me a long time to learn to trust first. I look back now and see how her persistence to be my friend and the sharing of deep fears and lies we tell ourselves was just as important as working out together or having our sons as friends.

We ran into others in the pool at the Norwich YMCA and made more swimming and triathlon friends. She invited her neighbor, who is a runner and triathlon volunteer, who wanted to get into the sport as well. We both worked to help her neighbor in the pool and at the lake to get her swimming. She also made the podium in her first triathlon.

We saw a couple of the guys training for a full Ironman, and they helped each other out. I loved the little community we were building. There were four of us women who became a core team. We would push each other in the pool, bike every Thursday night together, and teach each other new skills, like weightlifting, mountain biking, Spartan races, or scuba diving.

We put up with each other's quirks, like some over-communicating in group chats and others never communicating. Some of us overthinking and others calling us out on it. Some needing to make sure we knew the race course well and others just showing up. Two of the girls signed up for a half Ironman in Atlantic City, and one of them was so nervous she wanted to do the Sprint a few weeks before. At the very last minute, a month after appendix surgery, I went with her and raced in the Atlantic City Sprint Triathlon, and we had a blast.

We got ourselves a black leather string bracelet with a shiny, nickel-plated washer that said "Better Together," and eventually, we got T-shirts too. Sometimes, I worry that some of the others we work out with might feel left out, but I hope they know they are all part of "Better Together," even if they don't have a bracelet or a T-shirt.

We've done many fun things together, like running and biking in tutus or going on holiday runs. We still frequently meet on Thanksgiving morning for a run. I love the saying, "It takes a village to raise a child." It also takes a village to raise a triathlete. I'm proud to call these ladies friends.

I sometimes chuckle, thinking of this group of women like the motley crew in *Labyrinth*. They are my very own Ludo, Hoggle, Sir Didymus, and Ambrosius, each with their own strengths and parts to play in the march towards the castle. And even though it takes the group to reach the center of the labyrinth, Sarah alone must face the Goblin King in the end.

CHAPTER 48

Step Ahead and Lean In

*As Meryl Steep said but just two days ago, 'We have grown up learning to
speak the language of men, but now the time has come for them to learn the
language of women.' It's very simple, we have to choose to hold each other up.
We have to choose to have each others' back.*

–HANNAH WADDINGHAM AT *GLAMOUR UK*
WOMEN OF THE YEAR

A few years into working at Collins as the engineering manager and finally
feeling like I had arrived, I was awarded the STEP Ahead award. It was a big
ordeal where they flew women leaders to Washington, DC, for a weekend
seminar, including a panel review of women in the C-suite (CEO, COO,
CFO), classes on how to negotiate, and a gala.

Spouses and family were invited to the gala. My boss and HR flew down.
We got nighttime tours of the museums. It was amazing. Mike had never
been to DC, so he came with me and thoroughly enjoyed the event.

During the seminar, the event's leader made a statement in the welcoming session. "There's a special place in hell for a woman who doesn't help
another woman," she said.

Oh, that hurt. I sank into my seat.

Shit, I thought. *Did I help any women? Had I hurt any? Had I only been self-serving so far in my life?*

I looked around the large ballroom with the white tablecloths. There were only water bottles left. Lunch had been served and taken away. Was anyone else sinking in their seat?

She said, "It's time to leave here and vow to help other women. We are the minority. You may have gotten here fighting tooth and nail, but it doesn't need to or have to be that way."

My heart swelled, and my eyes welled with tears. I made a vow to do something. I was willing to explore how I had helped or hadn't helped others. I was willing to step up.

I thought about the women at my work at Collins in Rome. Some had helped me. Some I had helped. But still, others were obviously fear driven and would rather backstab. I thought about the first woman I encountered at the Big Aerospace Company who looked me up and down. I felt like she automatically hated me and saw me as a threat. I had vowed to keep her at arm's length. I thought about the first girl I managed and may have helped, but I didn't do as much as I could have. I was cautious with her. I held back. I didn't encourage as much as I could have or should have.

I returned to work and contacted the local Girl Scout leader to set up a "Women in STEM" session. It was kind of a flop, but I kept trying. I wanted to set up a women's group at work, and at the same time, an executive woman who was running the business unit called a meeting with HR and a bunch of women and encouraged us to start a women's group. So, I volunteered to lead it. The timing was perfect. Afterward, she called and thanked me.

"Make sure and look out for the rest of the women in the shop," she said. "Especially those women on the floor with all those burly men."

I was surprised by her comment and laughed shakily.

We made our own agenda, had potlucks, and held "Introduce a Girl to Engineering" in person and once during COVID virtually. The group is still going, and I hope it continues.

Simultaneously, the same executive had also recommended a book called *Lean In* by Sheryl Sandberg, the COO of Meta. We bought a copy for the women's group and passed it around. It was an amazing book that talked significantly about women in the workplace, why the gender pay gap exists (spoiler alert—it's because we have babies, and even if we don't take any more than the prescribed maternity leave, it still leaves us behind), why we constantly feel the need to sit on the sidelines, why we don't claim our seat at the table, and why we always have imposter syndrome. I felt immensely validated and looked around at many other women I saw putting their head down to work, not collaborating well, and not wanting to stir the pot.

Don't lean in. Don't look.

Reading this book planted a seed. During COVID, when the topics of diversity, equity, and inclusion became center stage, I realized that my female counterparts at work had to yell to be heard. I find myself still yelling to this day when I really want my point to be heard.

Other changes I've encouraged or made around the workplace that have been difficult for me are signing my folks up for Better Allies weekly emails and encouraging everyone I know to do the same. I brought things up to my bosses (all male), like their interview panel being completely white male. And I've told senior executives that their interviewee list is, again, all white male. We used to call our headcount/resource planning "manpower," and I asked to change the name.

Once, when my boss gave gifts to the entire staff (who were all male), he awkwardly said, "Sorry about the Collins blanket. My wife picked it out, and it's probably not something you really want."

I pulled him aside and told him that it was incredibly horrifying to listen to that, especially being the only female in the room. This stuff happens almost daily. Just this year, I was gaslit/DARVO'd when I told a director something was happening. DARVO means Deny, Attack, Reverse Victim, and Offender.

Another great class Collins sent me to was a leadership course called "Geared for Success," which had a similar message—supporting each other and making positive assumptions. For example, if you have to lead a person who is notoriously late, assume they want to be a good worker and be curious about what's going on. Maybe they have a sick family member to take care of in the morning; maybe they're dealing with IBS. Don't assume they're lazy. Find out what's going on with them. Make positive assumptions, and get curious.

I learned this also from Brene Brown's books and interviews. Never assume someone's "dirty look" has anything to do with you. Maybe they have a gut ache. Maybe they're holding in a fart. This is also very similar to Jennifer McClean, who says, "People have really good reasons for doing what they do."

These great courses taught me that my motives haven't always been good. Exploring this history of myself and working on healing made me realize the errors of my ways. I have been quiet to the point of being rude. I have been focused on my work to the point of ignoring people. I have been short in my text response to the point of probably losing some friends. I may not have been invited to that wedding because my quietness was interpreted as rudeness. When, really, I was expecting that person to climb my walls, and when they didn't, I deemed that they weren't a real friend. They had no idea how much I actually cared about them, how I wished for them to be happy, and how I liked their spark and funniness. I've lost friends because of my insecurities. I was hurt that I wasn't invited because I care about them. I never really showed how I felt.

Express your compliments, gratefulness, and your love frequently and often. People get hit by buses, choke on their breakfast, commit suicide, and can be gone in an instant. Don't regret not expressing how you feel. Because I'm short and to the point, I don't always express how I feel positively for someone. And I now notice the people in my life who do express themselves in that way, and I appreciate it. I have a couple of friends who text and are overly complimentary. If you've ever been to a 5k or any athletic event and you feel the cheering, they are like friends who are your personal cheerleaders. And I like that. And so, I've learned from them how to do that, too. It's taken a while. I can be a slow learner.

While all of this is great learning and progress, I still get the "waved hand" brushed off by men in meetings. I'm still frequently the only woman in the room, rallying and wrangling the team. They take it well, mostly because I don't make a point of it, but when the rubber hits the road, I still feel

THE BABE WITH THE POWER

that I get passed over for promotions and specific jobs.

I have learned that I have to lean into the conflict. Address it. This is not my strong suit. I'm typically so stunned that I never know what to say at the time. I have found that writing a response out and scheduling a meeting are important and necessary. Telling those folks how you feel may result in nothing, but maybe a tiny seed is planted so they change their behavior next time.

I do not think this will be resolved in my lifetime, but I'm so happy and grateful my company talks about it. We have Employee Resource Groups (ERGs) and Diversity Equity and Inclusion (DE&I) dialog sessions. We have reverse mentoring. I can suggest people get the weekly emails from Better Allies. I'm so happy I talk about this with other women, like my someday daughter-in-law, who is a doctor (and frequently assumed to be a nurse). We will fiercely have each other's backs.

CHAPTER 49

Docks

You make concessions … that you don't believe
you'll ever make when you're beginning.

—ANNA QUINDLEN, *ONE TRUE THING*

Mike and I bought a seasonal camp in the Adirondacks in Lake Pleasant, New York, around 2013. This camp was a 1957 trailer permanently settled on cinder blocks, with the side of the camper cut out and added onto with pine wood. The campground was situated at the south end of Lake Pleasant and had lake-right access with a nice sandy beach.

The campground had about forty sites, and we all shared two 100-foot, wooden-platformed, steel-framed docks. The campground renters, especially those with boats, were supposed to participate in the dock setup Memorial Day weekend and tear down Labor Day weekend. The first time we went down to the beach to help, the campground owner waved his hand at me.

"Only the men!" he called out.

My mouth dropped.

What is this, 1950? 1850? Do you know who I am? I am an engineer and former Civil Air Patrol. I do Triathlons and CrossFit. Who, exactly, are you speaking to? Should I put on my corset and get my parasol to watch this magnificent event of men carrying heavy things?

My mind raced with witty comebacks, but I kept my mouth shut.

Not only were women not allowed to help, but we were also expected to come down and watch, sit in camp chairs, corral the children, gossip, and gab.

The first year, I was flabbergasted. The second, furious. The third, fourth… acceptance. Finally, I was like FUCK THIS SHIT, and I disobeyed the campground owner and did it anyway. The docks were not that heavy. The men shooed me away, but I ignored them.

The feelings of disobedience and strength were a high. Until I turned around and saw all the faces of the women in horror. The three other men and I put one wooden dock down, and I turned back to get another. When I returned to the picnic table with all the other women, none spoke to me. I'd broken some sort of code. I was stuck in a time-warped age of patriarchy, and I didn't like it.

I realized that I can care about these people as humans and be kind, but I can still be myself and find the people who accept me for me. Those are my people. Strong women.

I do not submit to the patriarchy. I am not submissive to my husband. And I believe that all humans can do all things. But I can also be accepting and kind to those who are still stuck in another era. That's all they know. They are still kind and decent people. I originally wanted to throw them out with the bathwater. Sell camp. Leave. But I've come to accept the good with the bad. I've come to live in the contradiction.

I'm still stuck in a patriarchal marriage. I have assumed many traditional female roles, and it bothers me. Clean the counters, make meal decisions, clean the fridge, grocery shop, and make sure people are fed. But I also realize this is how I set things up. I take personal responsibility for that. It doesn't mean I can't change them, but if I gave up meal planning, I have a feeling I'd be eating a lot of shit I don't want to, like Hamburger Helper.

So, I stay the course and continue to support the local community-supported agriculture at Common Thread Farm in Hamilton. I continue to get my family to eat more plant-based foods. I continue to try to get three cups of veggies on the table.

And I continue to carry the docks.

Another Jagged Pill

For women to swallow
Accept
Take your punishment
Swallow
Take it
Suck it up buttercup
Be invisible
Be better than
Shut up and sit pretty
but not too pretty
perfect makeup
but not too much makeup
strong and drive your own career
but not that strong

CHAPTER 50

The End of the World

*Religions are like languages: no language is true or false; all languages are of
human origin; each language reflects and shapes the civilization that speaks
it; there are things you can say in one language that you cannot say or say as
well in another; and the more languages you speak, the more nuanced your
understanding of life becomes.*

–RABBI RAMI

I was always looking for proof of God. I know you're not supposed to, but
the blind faith of a childhood directive from my Catholic school nuns raised
a big red flag inside of me. One day, I found my own proof.

I was listening to a podcast called *The End of the World* by Josh Clark. It's
a ten-episode series on existential risk. Each episode deep-dives into one of
the risks that might kill us all. Pandemic, asteroids, AI, global warming, etc.
But the first episode starts with the atomic bomb scientists sitting around a
table talking about why we're alone in the world. They calculate the probability that the universe should be teeming with life. It's mathematically unusual
that we are here alone. It's like having one spore of mold on a piece of bread.

The government believed the probability of extraterrestrial life was so
high that they set up an organization and funded this search by scouring the

skies for radiation or signs of transmissions from civilizations. This organization is called Search for Extra Terrestrial Intelligence (SETI) and was later defunded, but exists today as a nonprofit. I remember that in the 1990s, you could sign up to let them use your computer for data analysis. They were scouring through so much data that they didn't have the computer power to reduce the data. They found nothing.

On the podcast, Josh continues to hypothesize that either 1) there must be a great filter that, A—we have not yet reached that will kill us off like it killed all other species off, or B—we already surpassed a great filter that explains why no other species exist in the Universe; or 2) there are already many other life forms, but they're protecting us until we mature, like keeping us in a zoo, or like the prime directive of *Star Trek*.

He explains that it could be that we already surpassed the great filter. Even though we know how to shock the primordial soup with electricity and create organic compounds that are the building blocks of life, we still do not know how they were built. It's like knowing how to make aluminum, yet still not knowing how to forge and pour it, or machine it to get a gearbox housing out of it. We still don't fully even understand how the precise molecular mechanisms of our genetic DNA in embryonic development signal which organs to be manufactured when. Maybe something in the human genome is a great filter we've already surpassed.

If we have already passed the great filter, and no other planet has species that have, that could explain why we are alone. So, that would mean that other planets might have life, such as animals and plants and single-celled organisms, but no intelligent life. Yet, we're learning that simple or non-intelligent life forms are more intelligent than we think. We're finding now that trees communicate with each other. We keep learning and uncovering more layers and more complexity, and it's all divinely juicy. The increasing knowledge and chaos prove entropy is real. So, this likely isn't the case because any life form likely would have evolved.

Josh goes on to explain that if our evolution/creation wasn't the great filter we overcame, there is a great filter to come. That's when he discusses the existential risks and deep-dives into each topic for each episode. At the end of the series, he circles back to the original topic.

Here's what I think is curious. Never once does he hypothesize that we may be divinely created. Even if he thinks in only scientific terms, you'd think he would have thrown that in there, even to poke fun. Doesn't that mean it's proof? Or does it mean that you could say the word "divine" is just another term for the items we have yet to describe by science? Like, maybe there's a third option, Josh, that we are our own creation. We have the power, and the ideas we keep coming up with are born of our own brains.

This theory all came together around the same time when I found Dr. Joe Dispenza. He is a chiropractor and triathlete who spontaneously healed himself after a severe bike accident in which four back doctors said he needed surgery. He healed himself with meditation (his own brain power). He vowed to study spontaneous healing if it worked, and so he did. He returned to school, learned all he could about neuroscience, and found cases of spontaneous healing.

What I liked about him was that he used a scientific approach. He took measurements of people's brainwaves, did the due diligence of a scientist, and came out the other side showing how to do something with the mind we'd call miraculous. Just the mind! He has numerous books and free YouTube videos, which I highly recommend. So, he's tapping into something we currently have no scientific name for. When our brains get into that deep meditation state, he says we're tapping into the divine, the Universe, what Abraham Hicks calls the Vortex.

I liked the term vortex because it's a mathematical singularity, like a tornado. I started meditating while visualizing a vortex in the shape of a tornado leaving my head, swirling very slowly, and containing all possibilities of the future. It doesn't just go to the clouds; it goes way out into space and to the end of the Universe. It represents the entire realm of possibilities. One where a tree falls on my house. One where I win the lottery. One where I live to 120, and one where I live to eighty-nine. One where I am fit and one where I am fat. All the possibilities.

I believe all the possibilities do exist.

Getting a speeding ticket, or not, when the cop pulls you over. A desire is like a rocket with a fishing line on it. A rocket of desire. I desire to be fit and win the lottery. Now, how do you know you hooked that possibility? When you can believe it, even if just for a second. Abraham says starting to believe is like hopping on the merry-go-round. Either you're on it, or you are not. And once you get on, you just need to stay on. Once you believe a little bit, you just have to nurture that belief. Dr. Joe Dispenza says that when you get to that spot, it's like hitting a golf ball into a sweet spot. You know you got it, and you want to get that feeling in meditation over and over. He went on to explain that's how he healed himself spontaneously.

For me, this brought Landmark, Project 42, and all the lessons I've learned together. It was the doorway into a spiritual life, a connection to the Universe that felt like I was in the driver's seat. Yet, there was more out there I could tap into.

I've seen this work over and over in my life. When things don't work out, I know I didn't believe. When I fail or forget to visualize a perfect future, it doesn't go as planned. For years, I didn't believe I could be thin or fit, so I didn't create a future that existed. Today, I visualize more adventure and book signing tours. My kids are happy and healthy. I've created vision boards, and when going back years later, realizing that it all came true. I've tapped into something that is currently unexplainable by today's science. Maybe today, I call it divine. Perhaps some say, "working with God." And someday, if science puts a name to it or experimentally proves it as quantum entanglement or string theory. I hypothesize science will explain it all someday entirely.

I realize a lot of people will have issues with this. There are still some who believe in creationism, that evolution doesn't exist. But I'd propose that divine intervention made evolution occur. I believe people who are already manipulating the timeline have tapped into that power, that maybe you call energy management, prayer, quantum entanglement.

Maybe it's just a different language that makes more sense to me. I have friends who are devout Catholics or Baptists, and they tout the light of Jesus and faith in God. Maybe it's the same thing? It doesn't matter what we call it; it's there. I believe it's there, and the words we use to define the belief are all just words. In the meantime, it feels a bit like magic. It feels like faith. It feels fun and lighthearted. That's what I want my spirituality to feel like.

I believe in science, and I believe in the divine. And I think they are the same. Science is just the descriptive terminology for what we used to call the unknown. We used to say the weather was due to Greek gods fighting, so can you jump on my merry-go-round with me?

Some people wear a cross to display their belief system, and I recently got a tattoo of the Fibonacci sequence. It's a mathematical formula describing a pattern that shows up from the shape of a galaxy to the shape of a snail. The sequence of numbers is found by adding the two numbers before it.

0,1 = 1

1,1 = 2

1,2 = 3

And when graphically displayed, it shows an ever-expanding spiral in perfect proportions to the bass clef, Mona Lisa, Milky Way galaxy, sea shells, maple leaves. It's pure. It's simple. It's my cross. It's my compass. It's my true north. It's a way for me to remember what was already there.

You are adored

What would it feel like to walk around feeling adored?

Knowing you were adored?

Who has adored you?

Have you ever adored someone else?

What a strange word.

Imagine the pet lying in a bed, and you look at it and adore it.

Imagine that pet is you.

Adore.

The Universe wants you to adore yourself and the rest of the world.

Adore.

What would it feel like if all of our belongings were adored? Taken
good care of. Clean.

What would it feel like if we adored our enemies?

Who would we be as a human species if adorement of all things,
plants, animals, and people were our only priority?

Imagine that.

CHAPTER 51

A New Earth

Spirituality equals the dedication to bringing the mind back to the present moment and slicing through the trance of my usual stories to the ground of goodness beneath them. Not a luxury. A necessity.

—GENEEN ROTH

While I had compartmentalized and defined my own view of spirituality, I still needed some day-to-day techniques that would help me cope with the ever-changing world, life stress, and whatnot. One random day, driving to work and fumbling with my phone to find something to listen to, I picked Oprah's *Super Soul Sunday* podcast. She had a six-part series on Eckhart Tolle's book *A New Earth*. I had read his book *The Power of Now*, but his teachings didn't sink in for me.

A New Earth was about to rattle my cage.

I listened to Oprah's six-part series and then got the book and read it. It would not have been as impactful if I had only read it, but listening to Oprah ask him questions and then reading the book drove it home. There are times when we're open to hearing something and other times when we're not. That's something to be curious about, too. I wonder if I had a bias previously. I think I did because my mom recommended *The Power of Now*, and

I was like, "Yeah, yeah," waving my hand.

I was ready to hear this now. I was ready to absorb. I heard him tell his story of great pain in his life to the point where he was suicidal. He then had a groundbreaking moment where he realized it was all bullshit, his mental state was all his own doing, and he didn't have to do it anymore. When he awoke to the fallacy of his story, he was sitting on a park bench in awe of the miracle of life. And he developed and devoted his practice to the power of now.

He also introduced the concept of the pain body. This is essentially old trauma locked in the body that is reactivated every time you are put in a similar situation. This was a huge a-ha for me. This! This was why I was "so sensitive" that I always "overreacted." Any time you overreact, you are reactivating an old pain. The response is disproportionate because of the accumulated pain, not the current pain. I thought about my need to escape. What and where might that have come from? And I started to write this book. I'd healed some old wounds, but I knew I had more to heal.

This "coming into the present moment" is now my mainstay. There is no escape. Escaping into food, running away, changing jobs, working out—they're all ways to ignore the present moment. It is a way to stuff it down, not face it. All I have to do is sit here in this moment and really feel the feelings, accept them over and over and over.

And in the moment, getting into a flow state, mediation, praying, whatever you call it, you can build a beautiful future. Daydream. Find the sparkle of the stillness of the trees or the wind blowing. Shining light and looking at what is, getting curious about my emotions. Not acting defensive, but when feeling defensive asking, *In what way, and for what deep-down reason, might I be defensive here?*

In his book, Eckhart also explained how he struggled with religion, and it wasn't until after this almost-suicidal-turned-sparkling-light shift in himself that he picked up the Bible again, started reading it, and found some fundamental truths.

"I am the light of the world. Whoever follows me will never walk in darkness, but will have the light of life." John 8:12.

What if it's all just symbolism? What if it's not literal? What if I always took the Bible as literal, and it didn't make sense to me, but it's all just symbolic? This makes so much more sense to me. But the "Lord" and the patriarchal nature still do not, and so, the words I choose might be different. I choose the word Universe over God, and I choose Light over Jesus. No pronouns, please. I'm going to stay off my knees, both physically and metaphorically.

Despite all of this beautiful learning, I still have trauma to heal. I still get overwhelmed. I still get the hamster wheel feeling of "it's a lot." Doing all the things right at work, doing all the things right as a mom, as a daughter, as a wife, as a neighbor, as a friend. Buy the mums and the pumpkins, prepare the baked goods, but don't eat sugar. All the contradictions. And I stop the rambling complaining. Never criticize, condemn, or complain. I can feel lost. And then I use this technique from Eckhart and so many before him.

Get in the present, breathe. Feel this arm, then the next. Listen to the sounds of the house.

Be in this moment, in this life, that I made.

Judy

The have to
The enjoyment
The drive
The obligation to perform
The have to
The obligation to use your talents for the masses
The feeding on
The feeding of recognition
"the bastards, they run this business," she says
and "of course it's your fault"
It's no different here, Judy
Here, there, and everywhere
Bastards
Oh, Judy
You are magnificent and
perfect, and I'm so sorry
Bastards
I still believe in the show, too

CHAPTER 52

You Really Don't Hate Me

You do not have to be good. You do not have to walk on your knees
for a hundred miles through the desert, repenting. You only have to let
the soft animal of your body love what it loves.

–MARY OLIVER

Life was getting better. My career was good, and I was consistently exercising and going to therapy. The kids were coming into their own, playing all the sports, figuring out who they were.

Mat had started dating a girl, Megan, who he had known in high school and who was going to medical school. I love to see Megan with Mat because she makes him happy, and he makes her happy. That's all a parent could want. We immediately pulled her into our family, and they even lived with us briefly. I asked Mike and Andrew to bike across New York on the guided tour, Cycle the Erie Canal, and then Mat and Megan did it with us the next year. Robert was still a little too small to do that distance, but he still wants to do it with us someday.

Mat and Megan lived in West Virginia while she was at medical school, and they would frequently come home. They came up for a visit one weekend, and my mom invited them over. They saw other people, too, and I was jealous that we didn't get to see them. The old wound of "everybody hates you" got picked open.

See? Everyone hates you, Joyel. My mind ranted and raved.

I didn't use the tools I knew. I didn't settle, find the feelings, and realize that an old pain body was broken open. I guilt-texted them instead. I said they might hate me, but Mike did nothing wrong, and they should come over to see him. I immediately knew what I had done and that it was wrong. I was ashamed. It was the same guilt that was placed upon me 1,000 times over. It wasn't even about them; it was about my old wound being picked open.

I cherish my kids so much and vowed I would never do this to them. That I would love them unconditionally, even if that meant they got a tattoo I didn't like or wanted to spend time with other people. I would gush love at them no matter what.

I immediately apologized, and we talked it out sitting on the deck in the sunshine. While the tension that day didn't entirely dissipate, today, we laugh about it, and I can joke about how ridiculous my reaction was.

I knew I couldn't rely on this wall I built anymore. I knew it was finally taken down. I knew this one fight was over.

PART 6

Triumph

CHAPTER 53

You Have No Power Over Me

I wish I'd had more knowledge before I started swallowing their crap.

–EMMA THOMPSON

I had gone to bariatric surgery consults three times. Once in 2006, once in 2014, and the last time in 2021. I had done a lot of research and realized that my years of excessive eating had spiked my ghrelin hormone (hunger hormone) production significantly. My doctor said the surgery would, without a doubt, extend my lifespan.

I gathered stories from as many people as I could about the surgery—strangers on the internet, people who'd done it and then completed Ironman, locals in my community. I sought out one girl who did pedicures and booked with her just so I could talk to her. As helpful as all the information was, ultimately, it was time for me to decide. It was time to own and listen to myself.

I knew I wanted this. I knew it was the right path in 2006 and 2014, but I didn't do it then because I listened to the coaches and others who said there was no way I'd ever do an Ironman if I did the surgery. I didn't believe that, but even if it were true, I was tired of the struggle, and I wanted this pain to be over with. I knew the surgery was the shock I needed to rewire my brain signals and my hunger hormones.

To be honest, I did not want to write about my having surgery in this book. I was incredibly afraid of the world's judgment, but I realized transparency was more important. This is what worked for me. I had tried all the other things—the shots, the pills, the juice fasts, the therapy, the alternative therapies, the pure fasting (that worked the best), and every diet out there. This surgery works, but you still have to put in the work. Its largest medical impact is in the first year, after that, it's all you. You can put the weight back on, as many people do.

Once I decided to move forward with the procedure, the relief came. I've realized that's a clue that it's the right choice. I was tired of listening to everyone who told me not to do this. The triathlon coaches who said I could kiss Ironman goodbye because I wouldn't be able to eat what I needed to train. The gym coaches who said that I wouldn't be able to eat enough protein. I was done listening to people who really had no idea about what the surgery actually was.

I was happy that I was listening to myself for what felt like the first time. I didn't realize what power I already had. I didn't realize these people had no power over me.

The pre-work for the surgery is extensive. It takes a year. You have to go to therapy, get a psych consult, gallbladder testing, an EKG, and other tests to make sure you'll come through the procedure okay. You also have to lose ten percent of your excess weight yourself. I was at 290 pounds at the start.

Even though I have had success with the surgery, I've hit many plateaus, so I still try not to concern myself with the scale too much. Focusing on the scale messes up my head. Some days, I feel fantastic, and it's up a couple of pounds. On other days, I feel enormous, like I never had the surgery, and the scale says I'm stable or down some. I've had days where I swear I'm the same weight as when I started and other days where I feel lean and like I'm running a four-minute mile, and the scale could be the same.

Most importantly, I learned I'm not a project that needs fixing. I'm whole and complete exactly as I am, and moving forward from that place helps me keep my head on straight. Regarding food, I learned to eat my protein first, whole foods, and not too much fat. I no longer anxiously search for the next diet or workout plan to fix myself. I still catch myself in this old thinking pattern—*Oh, I should cook rice, chicken, and broccoli today.* I stop. I question why. I ask myself if my body is genuinely craving a bland detox or if it is the old thought, *I'm too fat, and I need to get in control.* It's usually the latter, but I take it as a signal to maybe cut back on the fat/oils/avocado/etc that day. My body is signaling something.

Today, I work out for fun and to keep my body mobile. Mobility and health, in the long run, are the most important thing. I like setting new physical goals and am still chasing old ones. Sometimes, I don't want to do the workout, but I'm excited about the future goal, and that is enough. It's human nature to want to stay stagnant. To protect and preserve the energy we have. But it's important to push past that. And I think of the Sally McRae mantra, "Something is better than nothing, and done is better than perfect." Today, I'm training for the half Ironman, and next year, I plan to sign up for the full Ironman and obtain that redemption. I still want to be able to do pull-ups and run under a ten-minute mile, and I know it will come. After Ironman and after I retire, I want to teach yoga dance. And I know it will come.

I've rarely ever regretted a workout or its length or duration. I know there are times when I'm tired or coming down with a cold, but usually, if I push through or rally, I always feel better afterward. There are no bad workouts. Sometimes I cut it short, and I know I made the right choice. And there are times when I cut it short, and I think I cheated myself. It's a fine line of balance. But when I treat my workouts like play, fun, field trip day, or the swing set, it follows joy, and I know it's right.

Let that girl play.

CHAPTER 54

Joy Seeking

Oh you know, just another day on earth in the Universe, without having any idea how I got here. Just another day piloting this absolute miracle of a meat suit. Just another day full of endless infinite positive things to focus on and to feel good about. And to feel the Universal ripple of what happens when you keep paying attention to things that make you feel good.
It's limitless.
Great job everybody.

—SEBASTIAN SCALES

During the full COVID shutdown, we tried to keep in touch with friends with wine tastings and games via Zoom. One time, a friend mentioned she did the same with her high school group of girls who usually meet once a year. A friend of hers mentioned she was going to attend a virtual retreat with a woman named Lacy Young. Lacy had a meditation app and hosted Shift Retreats.

I found the friend of the friend on Instagram and listened to her interviews of other people and woman-owned businesses expressing their success with Lacy, and I was very interested. Lacy's Instagram profile read, "Guide for the high-achieving woman who desires an intentional, beautiful life."

Um, sign me up! I thought.

One weekend, at home, sending the boys to camp, lighting candles, and taking me time? I was in. I signed up for the virtual retreat.

Lacy had two pre-work courses to complete online before the virtual retreat. One was on your current beliefs. Writing down all the limiting beliefs I still had was eye-opening. I believed life was hard and chaotic, that I didn't do enough, that I had to do the "have-to" things before taking care of myself, and that I struggled with food. I saw how they were all just beliefs that I could change.

She also required us to fill out a form stating our intentions.

What did I want to focus on? I mulled it over. *I have a good job, enough money, a stable, hardworking husband, and happy and healthy kids. What's left?*

I didn't know if I should go back out for Ironman. I still didn't feel in control of my food. I wasn't happy with the amount I drank—not daily, but it felt like another escape hatch. Deep down, I still felt an unsettled unhappiness that I carried around for who-knows-what reason. And my origins and my feeling of being inherently evil were still not settled. I realized through that exercise that I had a lot of work left to do.

Her retreat theme was about finding and seeking joy, and we had to write about that word—joy. I curled my lip. I didn't like that word because it reminded me of my name. My mother named me Joyel because when she was pregnant with me and in the hospital with preeclampsia, she was watching a soap opera where a couple had a baby and named it Joyel. Joy for all the joy and L for all the love. (Feel free to mentally insert a puke emoji.)

People always mispronounce my name. My mom was going to hyphenate it Joy-el, but decided not to. So, when we had to write about how we felt about this word, I had negative connotations. Or I thought about the Christmas song "Joy to the World." It wasn't about happiness or bliss. I was going to change that on this retreat.

I set up the dining room as my meditation room for the weekend. I brought in all the throw pillows, bean bag chairs, blankets, and candles in the house and put them all over the floor. I set up a tapestry on the wall for a beautiful background. Somehow, I knew this would be special.

The retreat agenda was set up so that we did some talking and learning, then mediation, followed by journal time and sharing, then a break, and repeat. Two of the meditations were impactful for me. The first was the forty-five-minute ananda mandala (you can find it on YouTube). It made my dog go crazy and caused the power to go out, and somehow, this forty-five minutes went by like forty-five seconds.

The other impactful meditation was a Lacy guided transmuting fire meditation. I visualized putting my self-doubt, people I felt were overly critical of me, and my food obsession into the fire, melting like a candle and transmuting to crystals. I visualized myself at this fire outside on the grounds at Kripalu. The flame was as big as a bus. I was wearing a spaghetti strap shirt with no bra, dancing like a wild woman.

I am that wild woman.

A few months later, I met with Lacy one-on-one. I had signed up for a three-month session of Soul Care, where we would meet once a month. In our first session, I sat in my bed perched up (the only room in the house where I could close the door and make sure the family and pets knew I was unavailable) with a white plastic laundry basket flipped upside down to sit my laptop on, the power cord stretched across the room. I signed into Zoom to meet Lacy one-on-one for the first time.

It felt like therapy in a greenhouse. I don't want to discount any therapist; all my therapists have been great. Maybe I was just ready to move forward a little faster. But working with Lacy made a more significant shift in my healing than anyone else ever had.

For example, a previous therapist would say, "Self-care is huge; it's really important." But she didn't recognize that I didn't even know what that meant. I envisioned self-care as a physical, bodily "have-to," like the obligation to pluck my eyebrows for social and cultural expectations. Spending time preening myself was not fun or filling my cup in any way, so I always did the bare minimum. I would go from swim to work with wet hair—not straightened, moused, sprayed, etc. Bare-bones, shampoo-and-conditioner, towel-dry, up-in-a-bun wet. And what's worse, I felt guilty about it.

Lacy recognized this and taught me to accept and love what I do. Own it. Be okay with who I am in every decision that I make. She taught me that self-care is taking care of my energy and saying no to being around people who don't make me feel good. That wanting to swim and go to work with wet hair is okay. Wanting to do the things I want to do is okay. No guilt. No shame. Self-care is about taking a nap when you need it, feeding your body well, moving because you feel better, and going into the woods when you need it. Self-care is like Grechin Rubin states—treat yourself like a toddler. Do I need a nap? Water? Food? Quiet? Play? Self-care is also about not depriving myself of what I really want. This is following and seeking joy. Joy and self-care are intertwined.

I explained to Lacy how I felt at Kripalu—whole, at peace—and how I wanted that all the time. At Kripalu, I am kind to myself, I am grateful, I move my body with ease, and I don't overeat. There's no rushing or thinking about the next thing I have to do. I am one hundred percent self-care (ding ding ding…we have a winner). I write, and I find the flairs of emotion. Ding ding ding—self-care.

I came to the giant realization that my day-to-day roles as a mom, daughter, wife, and engineer have nothing to do with self-care. That the me who tries to be skinny and fit into the mold of society has nothing to do with self-care.

At Kripalu, I give myself permission to do the things I want and, more importantly, need. I move my body. I eat healthy. And I move my body because I want to, not because I should. I am confident in my choices. I have no regrets, and there are no shoulds.

At home, I am blue and heavy. I am mostly loving and kind to my family, but I am not always at peace. I am serious (like my grandpa), focused on the next thing I have to do, on the hamster wheel of obligation. I don't do what I necessarily want or need to do. I am not even ten percent self-care. I am maybe thirty percent healthy, and I am rarely confident in my choices. I'm always second-guessing work decisions and shoulding myself at home. I have daily regrets.

With Lacy's help, I healed old trauma, like forgiving Ann. Ann and I are still friends. The forgiveness is unspoken, but it is there. We are the oldest and dearest friends. When her mother died, I was there. When our close group of friends wanted to go to the high school reunion, we went. We send birthday texts, she comes out to visit, and I go there to visit occasionally. I will be forever grateful for the immensely fun childhood memories of swimming, playing games in the basement, going to air shows with her dad, and talking about music. In the present moment, any pain is lost, and I have found a friend who was there all along. Lacy taught me how to fully take those cinder blocks down and use them to build a new staircase.

We explored the energy of my dad and my feelings of being inherently evil. We went deep. We stuck with it. Journaling, writing, meditating. We kept it in plain sight and mulled it over until I was ready to spit it out and finally let it go. The wanting of someone I could never know or have. And the wanting to know who he was so I could hate him for his evil. But I released it all.

I forgave him.

And the hate was all gone.

Hawaii

It
Comes in waves
The feeling of needing sun and darkness
It comes in waves
People and alone time
Discipline and letting loose
Fun and work
Hard and softness
Consumption and fasting
I want it all and I want and need for nothing
Hoarding and purging
It comes in waves and the waves are big
Twenty-five-foot waves of fun
They don't feel so big the further from shore
It comes in waves
I need the dark right now
No sun
Alone
No people
It comes in waves
Rest and working hard
Hard work pumps out of me and there seems to be no rest
But the wave will hit
It comes in waves
Burning and numbness
Presence and distraction

CHAPTER 55

Fiercely Independent

To say what you feel is to dig your own grave.

–SINEAD O'CONNOR

While snowmobiling, you spend a lot of time in your helmet talking to yourself, thinking, zoning out, and paying attention to difficult terrain so you can navigate the machine properly. I might sing to myself, make jokes and crack myself up, or get deeply philosophical. Or every time I turn right, I might think to myself or say aloud, "Right turn, Clyde." The independence and meditative state is something I love about snowmobiling.

It was 2022, and I was on a trip with a bunch of good riders who were early to rise and not too rambunctious. Even though I chose this group, in the middle of the trip, I felt an immediate need to be alone. I thought of myself as a child and how, even in my work, I thrive with alone time. I need it. I crave it. I felt alone in the chit-chat at the end of the day, at dinner, and at breakfast. The constant being with people was draining me, leaving me feeling empty.

On this particular morning, I went out to my snowmobile after breakfast ahead of folks, awaiting people. I'm typically the first one out there waiting, and it doesn't bother me. I love the quiet. The snow always provides extra soundproofing. There are no birds this time of year, so the quiet invokes a certain wild stillness. I wasn't annoyed that they were late. I was just waiting, patiently, in my own head.

There was tension in the air on this day. Some folks were nervous about driving the sleds across the lake. Snowmobiling across a lake gets some people anxious. There may be fourteen or twenty-five inches of ice, and an ice road trucker could go across, but sometimes the snow melts on the top and creates a slush, freaking people out. There are enough stories of drunk people driving into river inlets that are open water or people going onto lakes before there's enough ice to cause people to worry.

I had an immediate urge to leave and go off alone. I just want to go. I want to do my thing. I want to go both faster and slower whenever I want to. I want to be alone. I want to get up earlier, set off, and go 300 miles in one day. I want to do all the things. Maybe I was trying to escape the tension. (I personally like going over lakes.) And maybe I was feeling pressure to change the course we had planned to follow in order to accommodate the folks who didn't want to go across the lake. This was a guided trip, and I left the ultimate decision up to the guide. He chose to go over the lake.

We started crossing, and one person had a major breakdown. Another was pretty upset. I felt guilty for choosing this course and for not saying to the guide that it's okay to go the long way around. We finally made it across the lake after a long stop on the shore, and I felt myself curling inward, wrestling against this knowing that life is better together and yet feeling absolutely parched for time with just me.

This demand to be alone is a frequent occurrence. I worked very hard to discover where it comes from, why it's there, and what it is I really want. It's the toddler effect again. Overstimulated, over tired, over hungry, or all of the above. I just need and want alone time, and there's a million times in my life I've completely ignored that calling. Today, I can tell immediately. I come home from a visit with my mom, and I need ten minutes on my bed or the floor playing with the dog or cat. I return home from work, and even though I get almost an hour in the car alone, I need a few more minutes at home alone. I can and want to be alone much of the time.

It's an aspect of myself I look at often. I hold it in my hand and turn it over like a stone. Sometimes, I muse with my daughter-in-law, Megan, about why we are both like this. We often discuss how Mike and I are equally independent, how we both love that about ourselves and each other, and how the allowance to do what we want when we want makes us both feel whole. The obligation to be with people can overwhelm me, and I now know I need to carve out time for myself. The time for quiet. The time for rest.

While I realized in my triathlon training that we can, as humans, do great things together and are better together, there are times I need my independence. And, most importantly, there's only rightness in that.

While I know that my family and friends will always be there should I need them, it's all about listening to that little intuition, following the breadcrumbs of joy, allowing time for self-care. It took me a while to figure that out, but the puzzle feels solved. I accept what is and allow my higher self to guide me.

I embrace "better together" while still honoring "fiercely independent."

Fiercely Independent

I ride
Alone
No regrets
No obligation
No one relying on me
No one yelling at me
No one backstabbing me
No one asking me questions
No one disappointed in me
Or to cook them dinner
Or to wash the dishes
Or to do the laundry
I ride
Alone
"We live, as we dream, alone" plays in my head from the Gang of
    Four song
So ironic
I think of Mrs. Fina and *The Grapes of Wrath*
Individualism wellbeing is inherently tied to the wellbeing of the
    community
Well, we are screwed
Because the community is screwed already
More proof to be alone
Plan for the apocalypse
Do I have enough tomato seeds? Beeswax candles?
There was a time there were babies on my hips

And now they're grown, nearly all adults
Here I am, Alone
Just like I knew it would be
Showered them with as much love as I knew how to give and I knew
    they would leave and it's okay
And if the apocalypse happens, come home
And we will learn to trap animals for food and to grow tomatoes
But that may never happen
And then I'll be Alone
I prefer it this way
Alone
Next to my alone partner
Who quietly exists in his perfection
And our perfect independence
Alone
Fiercely

CHAPTER 56

Universal Sparkle

People say I'm crazy. I say thank you.

—JESSI COMBS

I sat at my friend Kay's kitchen table in an old farmhouse in Ithaca, New York. My other Kripalu yoga friend had made a trip up from DC to visit us, and we were laughing and chatting. It was year two of the COVID pandemic, and work was incredibly stressful, yet I was growing and healing in ways I never had with the help of Lacy.

Kay is a defense lawyer, and she was telling a story of how she had to question a twelve-year-old girl on the stand about witnessing a horrific incident.

"I was so worried about having to question this girl. I needed to poke holes in her story, but at the same time, I didn't want to upset this poor girl who had witnessed a life-altering event. I was dreading it for weeks," she confessed. "I didn't want her to have to relive the event and endure any more trauma. It would have been super easy to tear this girl's story apart and win the case. But I was consciously aware of my impact on her life."

This is why Kay is my friend.

I felt this sudden appreciation of the Universe winking, nodding. It was like the Universe was Hannibal in *The A-Team* saying, "I love when a plan comes together." It seemed to me that Kay was put in this place at this time to take care of this girl.

Kay finished the story, "After I questioned her, I heard her come out and say, 'That was easy,' and I felt immense relief."

Tears streamed down my face. "I feel like this is Universal Sparkle," I said.

Kay laughed at my lingo, but I kept going.

"No, really, I feel like you were meant for this position, this spot, this job, at this time, and even though it was tough, you did it; you succeeded with kindness and compassion."

We are all diamonds forged in heat, pressure, and time, sparkling in the dark sky. All we must do is follow our calling, our passion, our dreams, our desires, and our joy, and we will sparkle. All we must do is look up and see the sparkle and the sparkle in ourselves.

I know I have to look for the sparkles, in big things and everyday things. It's the knowing that Glennon Doyle talks about in *Untamed*. There is a chapter called "The Knowing" where she describes being in tune with God, the Universe, or whatever you call it. She got there by meditating in her closet for ten minutes a day until, about a month later, she got in touch with that.

Her wife said, "How do you know it's God and not just your intuition?"

"I don't," she replied, "but it feels different."

She explained that it feels like liquid gold is running inside of you. I've had that feeling in meditations mostly. With practice, she says she can now tap into the liquid gold, the universal sparkle, God, the Universe, whatever, at any time, like in a meeting while trying to make the right choice. It's rightness. It's in harmony with the flow. I get that, and it's the same thing Lacy taught me and teaches. Let it be easy. Let it be light. Follow the joy.

It's connected to God/Universe, following the joy that Lacy talks about. It's being grateful, feeling grateful. Feeling all of the feelings. Looking at them. Leaning into the conflict. Negotiating your career, building your fitness muscle. It's all of it, all of it wrapped up with a bow called life. In the present. Because it's a present. Getting good food, body movement daily, good rest, tuning into the Universe/God/the Vortex—whatever you call it. It's not yelling at the kids. It's talking kindly to people you're in conflict or tension with in a loving manner with hope for resolve. Can politicians do this too please?

It's a total and complete mindset—a mindset that I have control over. I have control of my mood, my disposition, how the day will go, how I want to behave and interact in the world.

I don't take offense because I know that's a pain body. It's an old wound, potentially not even mine, and one that I may still have to heal.

I am grateful. When I wake up, I first think, *Meditation.* I think it was Joe Dispenza (and Lacy who reminded me) that when you wake up, think, *RPM,* for "Rise, Pee, Meditate," and hydrate. I try to drink a bottle or half a bottle of water. I like Lauren Fleshman's meditation of visualizing myself as a giant screw twisting into the earth. I think about the sky and stars and align and ground myself. I notice my body. I do a few stretches.

Our dreams are gifts, and our visions of the future are the power of prophecy. We can and should control the future. What do you want to see happen? The light, like Jesus, like the lightness in my body, the light that I visualize healing my body (which always works), is a symbolic metaphor of goodness in the Universe.

The knowledge that we are one with the Universe. That we are made up of the same particles, oxygen molecules, electrons, and protons that could have been on the other side of the Universe at one time. That standing in our own self-righteousness about being on the black or white side of that piece of paper (or the side of pro-life or pro-choice, or the left or right) gets us nowhere. We need to be here, in the middle, seeing and knowing and understanding both sides exist. We are not black or white or male or female. We are all of them. All at once. We contain both male and female energies and can tap into them anytime if we let them in. We can feel what it's like to be on the other side at any time. Just get curious. Just ask.

We can be a Universal Sparkle (US). We can be US. For US.

If someone said to you, "All you have to do to be saved is to believe in the Lord our God, Jesus Christ," would you cringe? What if that was written differently? All you have to do is believe in yourself. Your confidence is the light of the world. Your peace is the peace you give to others. You need to take care of yourself in order to take care of the community. We need each other, and we need ourselves. Give yourself grace. Learn to extend that grace to everyone. Know your needs. How much sleep, alone time, connectedness, and contribution to society (work).

It's weird to try to write a memoir, to organize your life, to mull over every detail of your story. I've had quite a journey, quite a paradigm shift.

I came into this world feeling less than zero, and now I know I can be as big as the Universe. I learned how to build my own labyrinth of puzzles and solve and deconstruct those walls into a beautiful garden. As my mom said to me, I was a gift from God. My existence is no longer a scandal. But I wouldn't have known that unless I had taken that journey. A journey to come back full circle just to myself. To knowing that I've had it all along

It's a wonderful life twinkle.

It's a wonderful life, Twinkle.

It's a wonderful life, so twinkle.

CHAPTER 57

Reconciliation and Acceptance

[We] will emerge battled and beautiful

–AMANDA GORMAN

When I read Viola Davis's memoir *Finding Me*, she described how she felt about her little sister Danielle being born, and I pictured my mom. All Viola wanted to do was love and protect her sister. And I could feel those same words from my mom. And I know she tried. And just like Viola and Danielle, my mother could not protect me from all the things—my life, my grandmother, the mean boys, the mean girls, Sister Sheila, feeling alone and abandoned when she went to work, random people who made fun of me, the desperate feeling of wanting to fit in and belong somewhere, the horrible bosses and being a woman in a STEM field, the patriarchy, and my own actions.

No one in my family ever said anything mean to me. They could have said, "No one wanted you." They could have told me, "You're a mistake." But they didn't say any of that, and for some reason, I felt those words like they were screamed at me. I felt out of place. Wrong.

Maybe my grandparents had resentment that they had to house and feed me and my mom, or never got to fully retire and enjoy life. Maybe it was the huffy puffy response when I asked for a ride or asked for help. Maybe it was how I felt pawned off onto my Aunt Frannie and Aunt Ellie when my mom needed a break. Maybe it was the quiet disposition of my grandfather that made me feel alone when my mom left for work. I always thought of my grandpa as my best friend. He spent a lot of time and paid a lot of attention to me. He would play catch and teach me how to weed the garden. He drove me to the Amherst Clearfield swimming pool and to softball practices. But maybe deep down, he was tired and didn't want to have to raise another child. Not white, not dark, not girly enough, wanting to do all the boy things, and not fitting in. I didn't fit the mold; not one shape of me was correct.

My mother and I do talk now, now that I've learned how to have a conversation without blowing up and ending up crying without resolving anything. Many years later, after many conversations with my mom, I was surprised to hear that she wondered if it was the best choice to stay at home. I was probably at least forty when I heard her say that. It's funny to think of your parents as anything but all-knowing, the person you go to when you need answers, or help, or to know what to do next.

"I wonder if staying in that house was a mistake," she mused aloud.

"I don't know either mom. I'm not sure it would have changed anything actually," I answered, trying to make her feel better.

When I was little, I looked forward to my mom coming home from work. If I heard the door, I'd come running for a big hug. I'd cuddle with her on the couch. I'd pine for her. I'd look out the dining room window, pushing the curtain aside so that I could see the driveway, waiting for her car to come up the road and pull into the driveway. I'd wake her up by climbing into bed and lifting her eyelids. She was the one I called when I was in college and my windshield cracked.

"What do I do, Mom?"

And she'd walk me through the steps I needed to take

I was always grateful when she took Ann and me out for Chinese or to Clifton Hill. I was grateful when she made things fun, like playing Scrabble.

She has a way of talking to everyone. Making friends with the nurses, receptionist, and grocery clerk. She is almost always upbeat and friendly to all strangers. I was quietly waiting behind her. Shy and not smiling. She is incredibly generous, always paying for dinner and always giving money to me and the kids for no reason or small reasons. She is fun. She played card games with her friends, and later in life, she made up "Nana's Reindeer Games," which we play at Christmas time every year.

As I grew up, into my teenage years, I wanted nothing to do with her. I was annoyed she was constantly criticizing me. My dirty fingernails or knees, telling me I looked like a slob, or that I forgot to pick up my wet towel. I was annoyed when she asked me what was wrong.

"Ugh. Nothing. Leave me alone!"

If she pressed, it would end in screaming or crying or both. I used to joke that Grandpa probably would take out his hearing aids when we started screaming at each other.

I was incredibly annoyed when I felt like she didn't back me up when I told her Sister Sheila made me uncomfortable. I felt betrayed when she told her best friend about something I thought was private. All my mother wants is for me to be happy. And the fact that I wasn't most of my life was driving her nuts. And still does. She's a fixer. She's a people pleaser. She's a hover mother. She would do anything for me and my kids. During my break for independence, I pushed her away. I barely called her when I was at college. I was annoyed when she did call. I didn't want to be told what to do. I needed to find and learn how to trust my own internal instincts.

Yet, she is my mom.

I saw a girl on Instagram who was all-consumed with the death of her mom. She went through difficult grief and ended up doing grief counseling. She said in an interview, "My mom was my person," and I felt sad. I felt like my mom isn't really my person, and I kind of wish she was.

A Bad Moms Christmas is one of my favorite holiday movies, and I can relate to the relationships of all three mothers in that movie. One is super critical, controlling, and perfectionist. Another is obsessed with her daughter and wants to move in, but she has no boundaries with her. And the third is missing most of the time partying.

Here is a perfect example of our relationship. I'm forty-something years old, sitting in a parking lot of Kinny Drug on the phone, fighting with my mom. After Grandpa passed away and we sold the house in the Buffalo suburb, she'd moved to live five miles away in a nice apartment. My mom's health isn't very good, and she walks with a walker, so we needed to make sure she had a place to live that was flat. I do a lot of errands, and she also has people to do them for her. She has a lot of doctor appointments that I take her to, and others do, too. She's at the point now where she is not driving and is homebound most of the time.

So, we're fighting. I'm crying. She says I talk to her in a mean voice, and when other people call, I'm so pleasant and nice.

"That's fake mom. I'm real with you."

She says she doesn't want the real me. I argue the same thing back to her. I tell her she's mean and critical of me, of my tattoos, and never says anything to the grandkids about their tattoos. (She didn't talk to me for a week when I got my first, second, and third.)

"Well, they're kids, and it doesn't matter. You shouldn't be getting tattoos. They're ugly." She goes on, "I just want the best for you."

I scream back, "THIS IS ME!! This is who I am, and you're telling me to my face that you think I'm ugly. It's rude. It's mean. I just want you to love me for who I am, tattoos and all."

She basically argues back the same exact argument. "Well, this is my opinion! And why can't you just love me with this opinion and all!"

And I stop. I laugh.

"What are you laughing about?" she snips.

"We're both literally arguing the same thing."

We both want the other to love us in the way we need to be loved.

I asked her, "What do you need me to do to make you feel loved?"

She said she wants me to be sickly sweet to her all the time, even if it's a lie and it's fake.

I shake my head. "Okay, I can do that if you want."

She asked me what I wanted.

"Next tattoo, I want you to ask to see it, ask me what it means, ask if I'm happy. I don't need you to lie to me and tell me you like it when I know you don't. I just need you to do what you would do for the grandkids. And not be immature and ignore me and not talk to me for a week because you're mad."

And she said okay.

And so, today, I have to pep-talk myself when I see her so I can be the version of me she wants. I feel sad that she's in bad health. I want her to be vibrant and healthy, and she's not. It's difficult to watch. But I mentally prepare myself to be kind and sickly sweet and not to take offense at any controlling criticism of how I'm doing anything.

My mom can be stubborn, persnickety, impatient, loud, and dominate a conversation and your attention. She can be overly reactive to any form of criticism (as I once was). But she is my mom. She's still the person I call when I'm in trouble first. She knows when I'm not happy, and I know it's best to get it out—whatever I'm not happy about—which might be trouble at work or a project at home. It's best to get it all out; otherwise, she will assume it has something to do with her.

She always asks, "Are you mad at me? Did I do something wrong?"

I call her every day to check in and see how her day is. I can get annoyed when she's all talk and telling me painstaking details about things I don't care about. She watches the Yankees games and tells me all the details I don't care about, but I kindly pretend to be interested and pay attention. That's her love language.

I see her at least once a week. I have taken her with me to Kripalu. I tell her about sessions with Lacy and what I learned. I told her I saw my dead father's ghost. I read her this book. So I guess she is my person. She has my history. I told her I'm working on our generational trauma and healing it for her. She says her rosary when I get pulled over by a cop, and somehow, I never seem to get a speeding ticket. Her rosary is magic.

I went on a retreat with Lacy and a great group of women I didn't know before. I fell deeply in love with life while there. I returned from that retreat with the poem, "There She Is."

My mother said, "Oh, you came home with such joy in your heart."

And I felt her become at peace knowing I was at peace.

There She Is

You saw me. With the lead weighted x-ray vest and helped me re-
move it

You saw me. In the maroon cashmere shawl and took my photo so
beautifully

You saw me. In the terracotta streets of Bocairent, thirsty and
bought me water

You saw me. In deep yellow and you were right and write and write
in my color

You saw me. When you shared your Baba with me and her gold
bracelets and I told you about my Grandma K

You saw me. After you cleared when you ran into my bosom and I
kissed your golden hair

You saw me. Sleeping. Next to your green stuffie, you were quiet so
as not to wake me. Told me I was amazing and made me deeply
'adioth' laugh over and over again

You saw me. In my wholeness, always, and knew I deserved the
black boxed May Lindstrom youth serum and showed me I de-
serve all the things

You saw me. In the purple shawl and so I bought it and I'll have you
with me forever

You saw me. In my yoga dance and validated my teaching and I was
called to give you the white power purse

There she is

Like peeking out from behind the baby blanket

You saw me

And so many before have too

But I finally see

There she is

And I see you forever in the rainbow and white light

And my mom can finally sigh relief

The Power I Have

Through dangers untold and hardships unnumbered I have fought my way here to the castle beyond the Goblin City to take back the child you have stolen, for my will is as strong as yours and my kingdom as great. You have no power over me!

—SARAH IN *LABYRINTH*

In October 2024, I traveled to Spain for a writing retreat called Muse with Lacy and her sister Kayla. This book was in its "shitty first draft" stage with a different title and a long way from the final copy. I spent the days musing, and the title and theme came to me.

During this trip, I also said a final and lasting goodbye to my dad. I dreamt that I saw his ghost, and I finally let him go.

The days in Spain were beautiful, and the women I met will be in my heart forever.

When the retreat was over, I wanted to take two more days and explore Valencia. I was feeling incredibly whole, beautiful, and in my own skin. I booked a massage at my hotel and had no idea it would be the proof I needed to see and understand the depth of my power.

When I think back on that massage, I want to capture it all—his sneakers, the pressure he used, the way he smelled, his black curly hair falling on his face. I've had a thousand massages. Only one, or maybe two, other times have I been turned on, but I never did anything. Not a sigh, not a groan, not a rotation of the hips. I made sure that they never knew.

This time, though, I couldn't help it. I started to moan. And sigh. And when he massaged my hands, I squeezed his hand a little bit. My hips started to rotate.

He was entirely professional and just kept going like nothing was happening. I was on the verge of orgasm when, all of a sudden, I felt him shaking. His hands were on my ears, and I could feel how much they were trembling.

And I stopped. I woke up. I realized what I was doing to him, and I felt terrible.

I had no idea I could do that to a man. I realized that my femininity was a force over all men—men I work with, men I encounter. In their eyes, I am both a sex object and a mother, and I can be kind or mean, sexy or withholding, and the power is enormous.

Suddenly, I was Rebecca in *Ted Lasso* when she realized all her executive men are just four-year-old boys, hoping they don't get yelled at.

I used to crave male attention. I wanted personal trainers to tell me what to do, to lift this and run on the treadmill at this speed, and I wanted the kudos. I wanted the "good job." And now, I've come full circle.

In *Labyrinth*, I always wondered, Who is Jareth? Who is his mother? What is he to Sarah? Are they in love? Is he just a father figure? Was she in love with him? Was she just tangled up? I saw him in her bedroom as a toy, and I thought, what toy would he be? Is she Eve, and is he the serpent in the garden of good and evil? Is he God? Is he the devil? Is he Sarah's demon? Is he Sarah's God? Is he the patriarchy? A symbol of all men—fathers and lovers, God and Jesus, all wrapped up into one?

He was the one who feared she would walk away, and so he held fake power. A power that never existed.

There is that scene in *Labyrinth* where Sarah enters the castle beyond the Goblin City and gives the speech to Jareth, the speech where she proclaims, "You have no power over me." If he is a made-up figment of her imagination where he held the power, what power was she giving away? She had to take the journey to figure out that she had the power, that she was giving it away, and that it was time to take it back.

All along, I thought my power was outside of me.

I think back to that day when my mom showed me that birth certificate. That gaping blank spot. My life has been lived in that blank. This life. This imperfect, tortured, triumphant, beautiful life.

All along, I thought I was searching for a father, but in reality, I was looking for myself. I craved to know the roots of my own roots, the heart of my own heart. Like Sarah, I had to learn to stop screaming, "It's not fair," and instead gaze into the mirror and see me—the babe with the power.

Ahhh. I think yes.

Ghost

Today is the day I saw
the face of Dad as a ghost
He has my eyes
He was pretty ordinary
He wore a light blue button-down shirt
He was bald with black
curly hair on the sides of his head
He looked like a dad
Long in the face
He was shorter than I expected
Thick
Solid
I didn't hug him
I asked, "What the fuck are you doing here?"
I just stared
Long in the face
Like a mirror
and my curiosity is satisfied
And it is done
As far away is the next galaxy or the star in the sky
from as far as all the rest of the people on this earth
You can go
I see no further need
This doesn't fill the gap,
the pining I had as a girl
wanting Bruce Willis from *Moonlighting* to be my dad or Richard

Chamberlain from *Thorn Birds*
This doesn't fix it
There will be no forgiveness
none needed
There will be no warm embrace
and so it is
it is done

To My Children

You should be celebrated for every aspect of your growth and your growing pains. You should be celebrated for your creativity, for your fearlessness, for your persistence and determination.

–RIHANNA

I am so, so, so proud of you. Way to be you. Keep being you. If I made any parenting choices that hurt you, I am so, so, so sorry. I think you know how much I love you, but just in case, here it is in writing. I love you to infinity and beyond. I love you so much, and my only frequent prayer/birthday wish/wish on a shooting star is that you are happy and healthy and live long, wonderful lives. I hope this book provided valuable information and a look into your history. I hope you didn't find it too embarrassing. I found these questions below online somewhere, and I wanted to answer them for you.

What is my happiest memory of you?

There are so many precious adventures with you. Of course holding you as a baby, falling asleep, cuddling, watching TV cuddling, Critz Farms yearly fall tradition, camping in Cranberry Lake, hiking, rock climbing, kayaking, playing games on the beach at camp, watching you play *Star Wars* with swords, Disney World, making Easter egg hunts (over and over again). Probably the happiest is Christmas mornings when you were young enough to play games, playing with the *Sponge Bob Square Pants* Legos, playing *Just Dance* with the Wii. It was calm. I felt whole. We had the whole day in our pjs to just be with each other. There were no have to's, no obligations. Nana and Grandpa came out, and we made a nice dinner.

Is there a want or wish for you?

For you to be happy with yourself and your life. I want you to feel whole. I want you to know how to process feelings. To feel all the feels; don't try to run away from them. The hard ones make you stronger. I want you to know you are whole and complete exactly as you are. I want you to feel that in your bones. I want you to be happy in whatever endeavor you set out to do, even if the endeavor causes pain, like an ultramarathon or something crazy. I want you to be safe and at peace. I want you to know how much I love you. And I hope you had the time of your life.

What are the best and worst parts about getting older?

The best is that I care less and less about what others think. I think caring about what others think is a survival mechanism. You need your boss to care about what you do, so you can get promoted and move up, but the older you get, you realize that there are less rungs of the ladder to climb, and maybe this spot on the ladder is just fine. The worst? The decay of the body. Keeping muscle tone and balance become a focus just to keep doing the things you want to do. And that's fine I guess; it's just more work than I thought it would be.

Acknowledgements

First I need to thank my editor, Kayla Floyd, without whom I would not have finished this book. Not only did she help me with the craft of writing and editing, but also provided constant encouragement to keep going. I cannot express enough thanks. Some sessions where I felt a mess and things were falling apart, you helped me to realize this is how it goes. This is totally normal. You are the BEST cheerleader, and I really, really needed that.

To Lacy Young, for showing me the way, introducing me to Kayla, and for all the love and meditations I know you've done for me. Your love is so abundant and clear, and I love you, too.

Thank you to my community of friends who would do anything to help me out, help take care of my mom, watch the animals, give rides to kids. My friends who will run with me at 6 a.m., just to keep me company and who will send photos of my kids in the newspaper. My friends who bring flowers to my mom when she's sick. You know who you are. I can't thank you all enough for all the love and support.

And lastly, most importantly, my family. Who has put up with my emotional rollercoaster throughout writing this book. Who is probably tired of listening to me talk about it. Who is always there for me for hugs, a shoulder to cry on, who look out for me. Who is like a rock and always there.

May we all continue to have strong love for each other.

Resources

Thinking of Suicide? Call or Text 988 or visit https://988lifeline.org/

Free mental health tests from Mental Health America at https://screening.mhanational.org/screening-tools/depression/

Women in STEM (WiSTEM) at womeninstem.org

Women MAKE Awards | The Manufacturing Institute (formerly the STEP Ahead Awards): Nominate someone at https://themanufacturinginstitute.org/women/wma/wma-awards/

www.geneenroth.com

https://rabbirami.oneriverfoundation.org

https://eckharttolle.com

Victim Mentality (Wikipedia):
Victim mentality is a psychological concept referring to a mindset in which a person, or group of people, tends to recognize or consider themselves a victim of the negative actions of others. In some cases, those with a victim mentality have in fact been the victim of wrongdoing by others or have otherwise suffered misfortune through no fault of their own. However, such

misfortune does not necessarily imply that one will respond by developing a pervasive and universal victim mentality where one frequently perceives oneself to be a victim. The term is also used in reference to the tendency for blaming one's misfortunes on somebody else's misdeeds, which is also referred to as victimism.

Victim Mentality: Definition, Causes, and Ways to Cope - Read the article at https://www.verywellmind.com/what-is-a-victim-mentality-5120615

Steps to overcome victimhood and take responsibility for your life:

1. Reflect on who you blame for what. Focusing only on one particular thing/instance/situation. Figure out who is to blame.

2. Understand what is to be healed. Seek out the inner child, the forgiveness, or what is to be healed.

3. Do the work: therapy, guided meditations to forgive, heal. Write a letter, write a book. Run. Scream. Process. Accept. Forgive yourself, too. Do not blame yourself. No shame or guilt.

4. Paradigm shift: Let the shift happen. It's not instant, but it can be. Practice gratitude for what is good.

5. Turn your focus outward and help someone out.

6. Give yourself kudos. Focus on what you have done to heal and give yourself a pat on the back.

About the Author

Joyel is an aeronautical engineer with several patents and published papers who has led engineering teams working in the aerospace field for over twenty-three years. This is her first personally published book, a memoir written to share her experience, strength, and hope for others who might have been in similar situations. She lives in Upstate New York with her husband, kids, dog, cat, and chickens.

Milton Keynes UK
Ingram Content Group UK Ltd.
UKHW041653151024
449742UK00004B/16